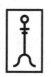

DR. ATKINS'
Quick & Easy
NEW DIET
COOKBOOK

COMPANION TO DR. ATKINS' NEW DIET REVOLUTION

Robert C. Atkins, M.D.,
and Veronica Atkins

A FIRESIDE BOOK
Published by Simon & Schuster
NEW YORK   LONDON   TORONTO   SYDNEY

FIRESIDE
Rockefeller Center
1230 Avenue of the Americas
New York, NY 10020

This Fireside Edition 2004

FIRESIDE and colophon are registered trademarks of Simon & Schuster, Inc.
For information regarding special discounts for bulk purchases,
please contact Simon & Schuster Special Sales at
1-800-456-6798 or business@simonandschuster.com.

Designed by Helene Berinsky

Manufactured in the United States of America

1   3   5   7   9   10   8   6   4   2

The Library of Congress has cataloged the hardcover edition as follows:
Atkins, Robert C.
Dr. Atkins' quick & easy new diet cookbook : companion to Dr. Atkins' new diet revolution /
Robert C. Atkins and Veronica Atkins.
p.   cm.
1. Reducing diets—Recipes. 2. Low-carbohydrate diet—Recipes.
I. Atkins, Veronica C. II. Title.
RM222.2 .A845 2004   641.5'635—dc22   2003065849

ISBN 0-7432-6000-7
0-7432-6646-3 (Pbk)

The information presented in this work is in no way intended as medical advice or as a substitute for medical counseling. The information should be used in conjunction with the guidance and care of your physician. Consult your physician before beginning this program as you would any weight-loss or weight-maintenance program. Your physician should be aware of all medical conditions that you may have as well as the medications and supplements you are taking. Those of you on diuretics or diabetes medications should proceed only under a doctor's supervision. As with any plan, the weight-loss phases of this nutritional plan should not be used by patients on dialysis or by pregnant or nursing women.

To my mother, Emma, who would have been very proud of me.
And, of course, to the memory of my dear husband, Robert,
without whom this book and the whole concept of
controlled carbohydrate fine cuisine would not have been possible.

—VERONICA ATKINS

ACKNOWLEDGMENTS

Very special thanks to . . .

My sister, Valentina Zimbalkin, whose culinary talents I have always admired and secretly envied.

My friend Anya Senoret, whose creativity extends from designing beautiful clothes to creating wonderful dishes.

Nena, who was visiting from Croatia while I originally developed these recipes.

My niece and nephew, Tina and Michael, who were my "official tasters" when they were ages eight and ten, respectively, and whose verdicts of "cool" and "awesome" were very encouraging.

My former roommate, Stella Siu, who gave me some wonderful pointers.

Kathleen Duffy Freud, Bettina Newman, and the late Michael Cohn, for their expertise and assistance in the original edition of this book.

Likewise, for the original edition, my editors at Simon & Schuster, Fred Hills and Sydny Miner, for their faith and support under daunting deadlines. For this edition, I thank senior editor Caroline Sutton, publisher Mark Gompertz, editor-in-chief Trish Todd, deputy publisher Chris Lloreda, publishing manager Debbie Model, publicity director Marcia Burch, and art director Cherlynne Li, among others.

All books are team projects. This new edition, produced by the staff at Atkins Health & Information Services, supervised by editorial director Olivia Bell Buehl, was no exception. Food editor Stephanie Nathanson worked tirelessly to make the second edition even better than the first one, collaborating with recipe developers Wendy Kalen, Cynthia DePersio, Grady Best, Mariann Sauvion, and Tracey Seaman. Nutritionists Colette Heimowitz, M.S., director of education and research, and Eva Katz, M.P.H., R.D., vetted all the recipes.

Without Erika Sommer, my writing partner, this book would not have been born.

I am also indebted to Nancy Hancock, who convinced Simon & Schuster that the original edition of this book "needed to be"!

Finally, I want to thank the more than one million Atkins followers who made the original edition of this book a bestseller, and who learned first-hand that it is possible to enjoy delectable food while following the Atkins Nutritional Approach™.

Veronica Atkins
January 2004

CONTENTS

PREFACE TO THE 2004 EDITION

Atkins Has Become Mainstream

In the seven years since this book was first published, many things have happened. Dr. Atkins, who pioneered the controlled carbohydrate lifestyle, died after a fall in April 2003. But his legacy lives on, growing stronger every day. At the time of his death, Dr. Atkins was finally beginning to see validation of his approach to weight control and overall good health appear in numerous research studies published in prestigious medical journals. In the months that followed, a flood of equally supportive studies has continued to appear—and be reported in the popular press—confirming the efficacy and safety of doing Atkins.

After more than thirty-five years of being considered controversial, the Atkins Nutritional Approach™ is moving into its rightful place in the mainstream. The last quarter of the twentieth century was dominated by the low-fat/low-calorie dietary culture—during which, not coincidentally, rates of overweight and obesity ballooned, along with an attendant rise in the incidence of Type 2 diabetes. It appears that in the first decade of the twenty-first century the tide has turned. More and more individuals are embracing the Atkins controlled carb lifestyle while bidding good-bye to their extra pounds.

The current excitement about Atkins makes it an appropriate time for this completely updated edition of *Dr. Atkins' Quick & Easy New Diet Cookbook*. This edition includes 50 new recipes to delight your taste buds. Among them are Almond French Toast, Quick-Grilled Chicken Caesar Salad, and Mediterranean Vegetable Soup. Many Atkins followers asked for more breakfast options, so we have created a section guaranteed to start your day right. (The names of the new recipes are listed in a different type-face at the beginning of each chapter.) We have reviewed all the recipes, making minor adjustments so they are easier to follow and the results even tastier. You'll also find updated nutritional information, including calories; grams of protein, fat, and fiber; total carbs; and Net Carbs.

Net Carbs are basically the grams of carbs that remain after you sub-tract the grams of fiber from the total carb count. Although fiber is a form of carbohydrate, it does not impact your blood glucose level the way sugar and most other carbohydrates do. Net Carbs are the only carbs that do af-fect blood sugar and the only ones you need to count when you do Atkins.

Finally, recipes are now coded to indicate the phases of Atkins for which they are suitable: Induction, Ongoing Weight Loss (OWL), Pre-Maintenance, and Lifetime Maintenance. In general, recipes that are ap-propriate for Induction contain no more than seven grams of Net Carbs per serving and do not contain fruit, fresh cheese, pasta, grains, starchy vegetables, nuts and seeds or their butters, or legumes. Those recipes that are suitable during OWL contain no more than 10 grams of Net Carbs and can include all cheeses, certain fruits, low carb pasta, and nuts and seeds and their butters. Recipes marked for Pre-Maintenance and Lifetime Maintenance may include previously restricted ingredients.

We believe that these enhancements make this book even more useful while you lose unwanted weight—and as you continue to control your carbs as a permanent lifestyle.

> Bon appétit!
> —Stephanie Nathanson, Food Editor,
> Atkins Health & Medical Information Services

LOSE WEIGHT, LOOK GREAT,
AND ENJOY YOUR FOOD

by Robert C. Atkins, M.D.

Like most people, you probably face a classic dilemma: You love food— and yet you either need to lose weight or want to maintain your present weight. Moreover, you love not just any food, but luscious, rich, satisfying food. Finally, you want to look and feel great while you eat well.

This can be a dilemma for individuals following a low-fat approach. But, fortunately, if you're one of the millions of people doing Atkins, you *can* have it both ways. Using this very special cookbook, food lovers will learn to create sumptuous dishes and control their weight while their calorie-counting friends look on enviously. You'll enjoy all the things that other weight-loss programs tell you to avoid. What's more, the recipes in this book have such universal appeal that you can serve them at a dinner party and no one will guess you're trying to slim down—unless, of course, you choose to share your "secret" with them.

The Atkins Nutritional Approach™ is not just another fad diet; instead, it is a four-phase program that becomes a permanent lifestyle based on eating natural, whole foods and avoiding sugar, bleached flour, and other refined carbohydrates, as well as the trans fats contained in most of the "junk" food on supermarket shelves.

Of course, those of you who have read my bestselling *Dr. Atkins' New Diet Revolution* and have tried the program know firsthand that what I say is true. For those of you who are not as familiar with it, the Atkins Nutritional Approach is specifically geared to correct the metabolic imbalance that causes people to become overweight.

Excess weight, especially a significant degree of it, represents an identifiable metabolic disorder called hyperinsulinism. Blood tests reveal whether you have it. And if you do, you can correct it—actually bypass it—by controlling your carbohydrate intake. The reason: Insulin floods the bloodstream only when excessive carbohydrates are consumed, so when you moderate your intake of carbohydrates—and focus on foods full of "good" carbs, such as vegetables, berries, seeds and nuts, and later whole grains, legumes, and other fruit—you completely skirt your insulin problem.

Getting your daily carbohydrate intake down to about 20 grams of Net Carbs (total grams of carbs minus grams of fiber), as you do in the first phase of Atkins, called Induction, will normalize your blood sugar, provide you with more energy, and keep you from experiencing cravings—all within two or three days. Because your appetite is so reduced, moderate portions will easily satisfy you. Simultaneously, you will start to lose weight—often at a rather rapid rate. And as a delightful side effect, you'll find the inches coming off just where you most want them to, in your waist, hips, and tummy.

For many years the low-fat doctrine held sway, becoming the standard American diet. But during the last twenty years Americans have gotten plumper. Although restaurant chefs, cookbook authors, and dietitians, among others, tried to convince us that a low-fat diet is, or can be made to be, satisfying, our stomachs told us otherwise. As a nation, we were always hungry, and in our desire to avoid fat, we turned to more and more high carbohydrate foods and snacks. Like the Chinese restaurant syndrome, we were hungry an hour later, meaning we ate still more high carb foods.

For any weight-loss program to be successful, it must be a lifetime eating plan. The metabolic imbalance leading to being overweight doesn't go away, so your way of eating must manage it forever. Other cookbooks expect you to live the rest of your life eating bland, fat-free foods. Their low-fat creations just don't work because natural fat creates, translates, and intensifies flavor, making you feel sated and full. Your body can't be fooled, nor can your taste buds. Imagine a life without butter, olive oil, cream, the crisp skin of roasted chicken, or a well-marbled steak. That is why so many other weight-loss programs fail. The requirements are so stringent and so boring that no one can bear to stay on them for long.

This book is designed to be your guide to a revolution in eating, what I call "a new diet revolution." Using the recipes in this extraordinary book, you will cook and enjoy eating dishes made of real foods created by my wife, Veronica. As someone who loves nothing more than a good meal, I am her greatest fan. Her recipes rival those of any restaurant or gourmet magazine. When you taste her creations, you will become fully aware of just what you have been missing. I love the fascinating paradox that food that helps you control your weight can be better, richer, and more sumptuous than most everyday foods.

Because sitting down to dinner together is precious time for any family, Veronica has ingeniously created mouthwatering meals that can be prepared in thirty minutes or less. This will allow you to focus on the good food and wonderful companionship when enjoying meals with your family and friends. That is what eating should really be about.

THE BEST FOOD YOU HAVE EVER TASTED

by Veronica Atkins

Dr. Robert C. Atkins and I developed this book not only to whet your appetite but also to give you the know-how to lead the controlled carbohydrate lifestyle. I never want you to feel as if you're on a restrictive program. Instead, you should enjoy the varied and luxurious cuisine that doing Atkins offers.

This book is also designed for the busy home cook, so all the recipes can be made in thirty minutes or less. These dishes are satisfying as well as delicious, nutritious as well as substantial, and easy to prepare as well as adaptable. In these recipes I did not skimp on flavors or ingredients because I didn't have to, and my sentiments about food would not allow me to.

Throughout my life, food has played a pivotal role. Growing up in postwar Europe, food was very scarce, but my family still enjoyed wonderfully creative dishes. As an opera singer I lived in many countries with unique culinary traditions and discovered many new foods and flavors. Then in the United States I met a kindred spirit, a pioneering doctor, who saw food as something much more powerful than mere sustenance.

My marriage and my work with Dr. Atkins and his revolutionary controlled carbohydrate program were a natural continuation of my lifelong love affair with food. I began to create low carbohydrate recipes that were uncomplicated and delicious. All of our friends asked me for my secrets. But when you're cooking the low carb way, you don't need a secret, complicated approach. Just a few simple steps can start you on the way to a healthy method of cooking for a lifetime.

You will be amazed how easy it is to modify your own recipes to create a low carb menu. Most main-course dishes are readily tailored for the Atkins way of eating because most of them are already protein-based. The recipes included in this book are some of my favorites, and after working with them, you will soon learn how to modify your own favorite main-course meals so they fit perfectly into your new controlled carb lifestyle.

Vegetable dishes are almost as easy to modify. Just keep handy a list of the acceptable vegetables while you are in the Induction phase. As you move through the three phases that culminate in Lifetime Maintenance, you will gradually add most foods back into your meals, although portions will be small and certain foods should be eaten only infrequently. The only foods that remain no-no's are sugar, bleached flour, trans fats (hydrogenated and partially hydrogenated oils), and other highly refined foods. I have also tried to make the vegetable dishes extra flavorful and luxurious, so they can even stand on their own as the centerpiece of a meal.

Breads and desserts are a bit harder to modify but not impossible. By testing different substitute ingredients, I have found the best combinations for creating delicious low carb baked goods. Fortunately, there are more low carb foods and ingredients than ever before, some made by our company, Atkins Nutritionals. Several of these are particularly suited to your baking needs.

Most important, this book isn't really about losing weight or even about maintaining your goal weight once you reach it. Instead, this book is about real food, sumptuous food. I encourage you to explore your palate, try new flavors, and see cooking as fun instead of a chore. The culinary arts have diminished in recent years, and because we are all so pressed for time, prepackaged foods wait on the shelves as a quick-fix answer. But a sea change is under way. People are demanding a change not just in taste but also in quality! They want foods that taste luxurious yet are good for them. The twenty-first century has ushered in the low carb revolution. It's also time for a renaissance in home cooking, and there is no cuisine more suitable than the kind that is appropriate for the Atkins Nutritional Approach™. This book will change your perception of cooking and weight control. You will come to view this eating style not as a "diet," which you go on and then get off, like a bus, but as a lifelong journey, and not as a painful experience but as a constant pleasure.

Quick & Easy Kitchen Strategies

When you cook every day, your kitchen has to be simple and well organized. And taking control of your pantry and refrigerator makes watching your weight much easier, too. The following are some practical suggestions to reprogram your kitchen for your controlled carb lifestyle.

Clean House

Get rid of the temptations! You probably have a lot of nutrient-empty carbs lurking in your kitchen: crackers, bread crumbs, potato chips, cookies, jams, and so forth. You don't have to throw them all away—others in your home may not be joining you on Atkins. The recipes in this book are appropriate for the whole family, but those consuming a higher level of carbs can add a few nutritious ones, such as more vegetables, whole-grain bread, brown rice, and the like, to the side of the main course you've prepared.

But do gather up these nutrient-deficient carbohydrate foods and put them in a separate part of your pantry and refrigerator. When you are cooking the recipes in this book, you want your shelves to be stocked with tasty, low carb foods. If all members of your household are doing Atkins, or you live alone, of course you can get rid of all those high carb temptations once and for all.

Managing Your Week

With a little planning you can whip up some simple building blocks for a week's worth of meals. If you prepare a few sauces on Sunday, when you're likely to have more free time, you can combine them with protein staples (chicken, beef, fish, and so on; see pages 209–210 for a complete list) or leftovers during the week. And you'll end up with a variety of flavorful dishes for those busy evenings. Of course, if you prefer, all of the sauces can be made when you need them.

For example, if you make Basil Pesto (page 161), you can serve it with grilled chicken the first day, use it in an omelet with mozzarella cheese the following day, and then add a tablespoon of it to your tuna salad on another day. So if you make a few sauces or dressings at the beginning of the week, your meals will be tasty and varied.

Shopping

At the base of the Atkins Nutritional Approach™ are fresh, wholesome ingredients, most of which you can purchase in your local supermarket. In fact, shopping for this lifestyle can make your visits to the supermarket shorter and simpler. In my experience, the fresh ingredients are usually found on the perimeter of the store, where meats, vegetables, and dairy are located. Always aim to purchase fresh, natural, unprocessed food; whenever possible, buy organic foods that are grown without hormones and pesticides. Once a month or so, you may need to go to a specialty- or natural-food store for specific ingredients. Depending on where you live, you may not be able to find some of the ingredients locally; however, most are available by mail order. Atkins Nutritionals offers many low carb products at www.atkins.com and in the printed catalog. (Call 1-800-6-ATKINS for a catalog.)

Equipment

A quick and easy kitchen should contain some time-saving and easy-to-use pieces of equipment. These few additions to your basic store of pots and pans can greatly reduce both preparation and cooking time.

FOOD PROCESSOR: A must for any kitchen, it allows you to create innumerable dishes and frees you from depending on bottled dressings, sauces, and canned soups.

RAMEKINS: Great for baking individual portions, ramekins are small dishes that are oven-safe and reduce cooking time, too.

FLAMEPROOF SKILLET: This flexible piece of cookware offers the convenience of transferring a dish directly from the stovetop to the oven, a must-have for creating a flawless frittata.

MUFFIN PANS: A carb-control aid, muffin pans provide built-in portion control and reduce the cooling time needed for quick breads.

IMMERSION BLENDER: This is the ideal tool for puréeing soups and sauces. Instead of transferring liquids to a blender, simply immerse the blending blade right in the pot or saucepan.

INSTANT-READ THERMOMETER: This tiny tool takes all the guesswork out of cooking protein foods. When you use temperature as your guide, you ensure that your food is cooked long enough to kill off microorganisms but not so long that it gets tough or dry.

HIDDEN CARBOHYDRATES

Not long ago it was hard to figure out the real carbohydrate content of many foods. But now, with labeling laws in place, the "carbohydrate grams per serving" is clearly shown on the Nutrition Facts label of all processed foods. In assessing carbohydrates, make sure you consider your serving size (usually shown on the top of the label). All too often the serving size, for which carbohydrate grams are measured, is only a small portion of the whole. This can be very misleading, so read all labels carefully. As a rule, when a label states that a portion is "less than 1 gram" of carbohydrate, count it as a full gram because it could be up to 0.99 percent of a gram. When it comes to counting carbohydrates, it's always better to overestimate.

Remember that when you do Atkins, the only carbs you need to count are Net Carbs, which you can calculate by subtracting grams of fiber from the total grams of carbohydrate. (See pages 7–8 for more on Net Carbs.)

You may be surprised by some foods in which carbohydrates lurk. Here are some you should watch out for:

- Luncheon meats, bottled salad dressings, imitation mayonnaise, ketchup, relish, pickles, and diet cheeses. These often have added sugars or starches.

- Prepared gravies and sauces. These often are thickened with starches, or sweetened with sugar or corn syrup.

- "Sugar-free" products. Products may not contain sugar but still have caloric sweeteners including corn syrup, cane syrup, date sugar, honey, and molasses. Check ingredients carefully.

- Dairy products. Remember that, as a rule, the lower the fat content of a milk product, the higher its carbohydrate grams. Cream is lower in carbs than skim milk; sour cream is lower than yogurt.
- Chewing gum, breath mints, cough drops, and cough syrups. These often contain sugar and carbohydrates.
- "Low-fat" and "fat-free" foods. Cutting fat usually means that more sugars and other carbohydrates have been added.

For a list of Atkins Nutritionals products that are included in recipes, turn to page 217. Atkins low carb alternative food products are available in grocery stores, natural-food stores, and many other outlets. Go to www. atkins.com to find a retailer near you.

Hints for Lowering the Carb Content of Other Recipes
- Refer to the Acceptable Foods list in the back of this book (pages 209–213) for information on foods you can eat on the Induction phase of Atkins.
- For dredging, use Atkins Quick Quisine™ Bake Mix, soy flour, tofu flour, or ground nuts or seeds instead of bleached flour.
- Use mashed cauliflower, not potatoes, to thicken sauces. And keep on hand a low carbohydrate thickener (such as ThickenThin™ Not Starch thickener).
- Yellow or white onions are higher in carbs than green onions (scallions); on Induction you may want to substitute green onions in small amounts or add a bit of onion powder instead.
- When a recipe contains several vegetables, refer to the list of Low Carbohydrate Vegetables (page 212). If you are on Induction or Ongoing Weight Loss, omit from the recipe vegetables that are not on the list and substitute those that are.
- Change the ratio of vegetables to protein. On Induction, cut back on the amount of vegetables and increase the amount of protein.
- In recipes that call for a topping of breading, use a mixture of finely chopped nuts and Atkins Quick Quisine™ Bake Mix. Or make your own crumbs from low carb bread.

- For spreads and dips, use elegant whole endive leaves, hard-boiled eggs, or plain frittatas, cut into wedges, instead of crackers and bread. Or use low carb breads and crackers.

- Most quiches and other baked egg dishes can be made without a crust. Just butter your pan well and pour the filling directly in it.

- Experiment with sugar substitutes. We recommend sucralose (marketed as Splenda®) or saccharin (marketed as Sweet'N Low®). Some other sweeteners lose their sweetness when heated.

QUICK & EASY GUIDE TO THE
QUICK & EASY NEW DIET COOKBOOK

This cookbook is a companion to *Dr. Atkins' New Diet Revolution,* which provides an in-depth explanation of the four phases of the Atkins Nutritional Approach™ and the scientific principles behind it. As you use this cookbook, keep in mind that your success at doing Atkins depends on accurately counting the total number of grams of Net Carbs you consume in a day. You should therefore determine how many Net Carbs you have in each meal; then, to ensure that you do not exceed your carb threshold, add in any additional carbs you consume in snacks or desserts. We have created recipes in this book that are appropriate for each phase of Atkins, and each recipe is designated for the phases for which it is suitable. Following are some brief guidelines to keep in mind when choosing a recipe.

- During *Induction,* you should consume no more than 20 grams of Net Carbs a day. In this phase, you eat primarily protein, natural fat, salad greens, and other low carb vegetables. But remember, you must follow this phase for only a minimum of two weeks. After two weeks you can choose to move to the next phase or stay with Induction if you have a lot of weight to lose.

- During *Ongoing Weight Loss,* you need to find your own Critical Carbohydrate Level for Losing (CCLL), as explained in *Dr. Atkins' New Diet Revolution.* You will gradually add back more low carb vegetables, berries, nuts, and seeds. Most people find that a level of 30 to 50 grams of Net Carbs each day is their CCLL.

- During *Pre-Maintenance,* weight loss is slowed considerably until you reach and then maintain your goal weight for at least a month. Most people are able to add back occasional and moderate portions of other fruits, whole grains, legumes, and starchy vegetables.
- During *Lifetime Maintenance,* you simply maintain your goal weight by continuing to control your consumption of carbs.

Don't forget to think in terms of total grams of Net Carbs per meal and per day. In Induction, most people find it helpful to aim for about 4 grams at breakfast, 5 at lunch, and 8 at dinner. This allows you the leeway to have a couple of low carb snacks between meals.

If you find our recipes as tasty and useful as we think you will, you will also enjoy the recipes in *Dr. Atkins' New Diet Revolution* and *Dr. Atkins' New Diet Cookbook.* The Atkins Web site is also always developing new recipes. Go to www.atkins.com, where you can also sign up for the bi-monthly electronic *Atkins Food & Recipe Newsletter.*

APPETIZERS

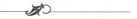

Smoked Salmon Rolls

Chicken Liver Pâté with Cloves

Deviled Eggs

Curried Stuffed Eggs

Baked Goat Cheese and Ricotta Custards

Zucchini Rolls with Chèvre

Artichoke Hearts Wrapped in Bacon

Guacamole

Savory Nut Mix

Marinated Mozzarella

Caponata and Goat Cheese Squares

SMOKED SALMON ROLLS

hese elegant hors d'oeuvres are delicate and flavorful. Serve them with a drizzle of lemon juice if desired.

PREP TIME: 10 MINUTES

4 SERVINGS

4 ounces thinly sliced smoked
   salmon
2 tablespoons Horseradish Cream
   (page 153)

1 tablespoon capers
1 teaspoon chopped fresh dill

1. Cut the salmon into 1-inch strips.

2. Put a small dollop of Horseradish Cream on one end of each salmon strip. Top with a caper and a sprinkling of dill.

3. Roll up the salmon strips jelly-roll style and secure with toothpicks. Serve immediately.

PER SERVING
carbs: 0 grams; Net Carbs: 0 grams;
fiber: 0 grams; protein: 5 grams; fat: 2.5 grams; calories: 47

PHASES 1–4

CHICKEN LIVER PÂTÉ WITH CLOVES

âté is a timeless, sophisticated hors d'oeuvre as well as a simple, delicious snack. Try it spooned into hard-boiled egg whites for a sumptuous twist on traditional deviled eggs.

PREP TIME: 15 MINUTES • COOK TIME: 10 MINUTES
4 SERVINGS (YIELD: ⅓ CUP)

½ pound chicken livers

2 tablespoons butter, softened

2 tablespoons grated onion

2 teaspoons dry sherry (optional)

¼ teaspoon dry mustard

⅛ teaspoon ground cloves

pinch of cayenne pepper

salt and pepper to taste

1. Place the chicken livers in a small saucepan. Add enough water to just cover, bring to a boil, and lower the heat. Simmer, covered, for 5–8 minutes, or until cooked through. Drain and transfer the livers to a food processor.

2. Add the butter, onion, sherry if using, mustard, cloves, cayenne, salt, and pepper. Purée, scraping down the sides of the food processor, until smooth, about 1 minute. Transfer the pâté to a serving bowl and refrigerate for 10 minutes. Serve immediately, or refrigerate, covered, for up to 3 days.

PER SERVING
carbs: 2.5 grams; Net Carbs: 2.5 grams;
fiber: 0 grams; protein: 10.5 grams; fat: 8 grams; calories: 125

PHASES 1–4

DEVILED EGGS

You can easily double or triple the recipe for these tangy stuffed eggs. When you serve a crowd, make extra—they'll disappear very quickly.

PREP TIME: 15 MINUTES • COOK TIME: 15 MINUTES
4 SERVINGS

4 hard-boiled eggs
1 tablespoon minced celery
1 tablespoon finely chopped
    scallion (white part only)
1 tablespoon mayonnaise
2 teaspoons drained nonpareil
    capers

½ teaspoon Dijon mustard
salt and pepper to taste
paprika and chopped fresh flat-leaf
    parsley or chopped fresh dill for
    garnish

1. Cut the eggs in half. With a spoon, scrape the yolks into a bowl. Reserve the white halves intact.

2. Add the celery, scallion, mayonnaise, capers, mustard, salt, and pepper to the egg yolks. Mix well.

3. Divide the yolk mixture evenly among the reserved whites, mounding it slightly. Garnish with paprika and parsley or dill if desired. Serve immediately, or refrigerate, covered, for up to 1 day.

PER SERVING
carbs: 1 gram; Net Carbs: 1 gram;
fiber: 0 grams; protein: 7.5 grams; fat: 8.5 grams; calories: 111

PHASES 1–4

CURRIED STUFFED EGGS

This deviled egg variation pairs well with cut-up vegetables, such as bell peppers, celery, radishes, and jicama.

PREP TIME: 15 MINUTES • COOK TIME: 15 MINUTES
4 SERVINGS

---

4 hard-boiled eggs

1 tablespoon mayonnaise

1 teaspoon Dijon mustard

½ teaspoon curry powder

pinch of cayenne pepper

salt and pepper to taste

1. Cut the eggs in half. With a spoon, scrape the yolks into a bowl. Reserve the white halves intact.

2. Add the mayonnaise, mustard, curry powder, cayenne, salt, and pepper to the egg yolks. Mix well.

3. Divide the yolk mixture evenly among the reserved whites, mounding it slightly. Serve immediately, or refrigerate, covered, for up to 1 day.

PER SERVING
carbs: 1 gram; Net Carbs: 1 gram;
fiber: 0 grams; protein: 6.5 grams; fat: 8 grams; calories: 105

PHASES 1–4

BAKED GOAT CHEESE
AND RICOTTA CUSTARDS

*S*avory custards wrapped in spinach leaves and then baked in individual ramekins make a terrific first course or luncheon entrée. Serve them on mixed greens.

PREP TIME: 20 MINUTES • BAKE TIME: 30 MINUTES
4 SERVINGS

butter for greasing the ramekins
1 cup whole-milk ricotta cheese
6 ounces fresh goat cheese
2 eggs, lightly beaten
3 tablespoons grated Parmesan
  cheese

3 tablespoons coarsely chopped
  walnuts
2 tablespoons chopped fresh basil
salt and pepper to taste
12 large spinach leaves, stemmed
  and washed

1. Preheat the oven to 350°F. Generously butter four 5-ounce ramekins.

2. Combine the ricotta, goat cheese, eggs, Parmesan, walnuts, basil, salt, and pepper. Mix well.

3. Line each ramekin with 3 spinach leaves. Add the cheese mixture to the ramekins, filling them ¾ full, and bake for 30 minutes. Let cool for 5 minutes.

4. To serve, place a small serving plate on top of each ramekin and turn the ramekin upside down, cutting away any spinach that overlaps the rim. Tap the bottom of each ramekin, then remove it, releasing the custard. The ramekin should slide off easily. Serve immediately.

PER SERVING
carbs: 4.5 grams; Net Carbs: 3.5 grams;
fiber: 1 gram; protein: 21 grams; fat: 24.5 grams; calories: 321

PHASES 2–4

ZUCCHINI ROLLS WITH CHÈVRE

You can substitute another soft cheese, such as cream cheese or ricotta, for the chèvre.

PREP TIME: 10 MINUTES • COOK TIME: 5 MINUTES
4 SERVINGS

1 large zucchini, cut lengthwise into eight ⅜-inch-thick slices
2 tablespoons olive oil
2 ounces chèvre cheese, softened

2 tablespoons chopped tomato
2 tablespoons chopped fresh flat-leaf parsley
salt and pepper to taste

1. Preheat the grill or broiler. Brush the zucchini slices with oil and grill or broil them for 2–3 minutes on each side, or until lightly browned. Let the zucchini cool slightly.

2. Spread each zucchini slice with 1½ teaspoons of chèvre. Top with 1 teaspoon of chopped tomato and 1 teaspoon of parsley, and season with salt and pepper.

3. Roll up the zucchini slices jelly-roll style and secure with toothpicks. Serve immediately.

PER SERVING
carbs: 3 grams; Net Carbs: 2 grams;
fiber: 1 gram; protein: 3.5 grams; fat: 10 grams; calories: 111

PHASES 1–4

Artichoke Hearts Wrapped in Bacon

You'll appreciate how easy and quick this two-ingredient hors d'oeuvre is to prepare when company drops by unexpectedly.

PREP TIME: 15 MINUTES • COOK TIME: 10 MINUTES
4 SERVINGS

½ pound thinly sliced bacon
two 14-ounce cans artichoke
    hearts, drained and halved, or
    one 10½-ounce package frozen
    artichoke hearts, thawed and
    halved

1. Preheat the broiler. Cut the bacon slices in half and place them on a baking sheet. Broil for 3 minutes. Let cool.
2. When the bacon is cool enough to handle, wrap each artichoke half in a piece of bacon, broiled side facing inward, and secure with a toothpick. Broil for 4–5 minutes, or until the bacon is brown and crisp. Serve immediately.

PER SERVING
carbs: 11.5 grams; Net Carbs: 2.5 grams;
fiber: 9 grams; protein: 10 grams; fat: 10 grams; calories: 164

PHASES 1–4

GUACAMOLE

*G*uacamole is not just a dip. The spicy Mexican specialty makes a tasty topping for an omelet or a colorful bed for grilled chicken.

PREP TIME: 15 MINUTES
4 SERVINGS

2 ripe Haas avocados, cut into
   small cubes

⅔ cup finely chopped onion

⅔ cup finely chopped tomato

½ jalapeño chili, finely chopped, or
   more to taste

5 tablespoons chopped fresh
   cilantro

2 tablespoons fresh lime juice

2 tablespoons olive oil

salt and pepper to taste

Combine all the ingredients in a bowl and mix gently. Serve immediately, or refrigerate, covered, for up to 2 days.

PER SERVING
carbs: 12 grams; Net Carbs: 6 grams;
fiber: 6 grams; protein: 3 grams; fat: 22.5 grams; calories: 242

PHASES 1–4

SAVORY NUT MIX

*F*lavored with butter and with a hint of heat and herbs, this addictive cocktail mix is a cinch to prepare.

PREP TIME: 10 MINUTES • COOK TIME: 15 MINUTES
10 SERVINGS

one 12-ounce can mixed dry-
   roasted salt-free cocktail nuts
4 cups popped popcorn
3 tablespoons butter, melted

2 teaspoons minced fresh thyme
1 teaspoon kosher salt
¼ teaspoon cayenne pepper
¼ teaspoon garlic powder

1. Preheat the oven to 275°F. In a large roasting pan, toss the nuts and popcorn with the butter. Sprinkle evenly with the thyme. Combine the salt, cayenne pepper, and garlic powder. Sprinkle it over the nut mixture and toss well.

2. Bake for 15 minutes. Transfer to a large sheet of wax paper and let cool. Store in an airtight container.

PER SERVING
carbs: 11 grams; Net Carbs: 7 grams;
fiber: 4 grams; protein: 6.5 grams; fat: 22 grams; calories: 255

PHASES 3 AND 4

MARINATED MOZZARELLA

Fresh mozzarella is sold in Italian delis and many supermarkets. If you can't find it, you can use the prepackaged kind sold in the dairy section.

PREP TIME: 10 MINUTES • MARINATE TIME: 2 HOURS
8 SERVINGS

½ cup extra-virgin olive oil

1 teaspoon minced fresh oregano

1 large clove garlic, minced

¼ teaspoon dried red pepper flakes

¼ teaspoon sweet paprika

1 pound fresh mozzarella cheese,
   cut into ¾-inch cubes

1. In a large, shallow dish, combine all the ingredients except the mozzarella.

2. Add the mozzarella and toss to coat. Let stand, covered, at room temperature for 2 hours before serving.

PER SERVING
carbs: 3 grams; Net Carbs: 3 grams;
fiber: 0 grams; protein: 7 grams; fat: 13.5 grams; calories: 162

PHASES 1–4

CAPONATA AND
GOAT CHEESE SQUARES

*P*iquant caponata (eggplant and olive spread) and mellow goat cheese are
a great flavor combination. Italian eggplant is milder than its larger cousin and
doesn't need to be salted before cooking.

PREP TIME: 10 MINUTES • COOK TIME: 10 MINUTES
4 SERVINGS

1 tablespoon olive oil

1 small Italian eggplant (about
    5 ounces), cut in ⅓-inch cubes

¼ cup oil-cured black olives, pitted
    and sliced

2 teaspoons tomato paste

1 teaspoon red wine vinegar

salt and pepper to taste

2 slices Atkins Bakery™ Ready-to-
    Eat Sliced White Bread, toasted

2 ounces goat cheese, cut into
    8 pieces

1. Heat the oil in a small skillet over medium heat. Add the eggplant
and cook for 5 minutes, or until softened. Add the olives, tomato paste, and
vinegar. Mix well and cook 5 minutes more. Add the salt and pepper. Let
cool to room temperature.

2. Preheat the broiler. Cut each slice of toast into 4 squares. Top each
square with ⅛ of the eggplant mixture and 1 piece of goat cheese. Place the
squares under the broiler for 20 seconds, just until the cheese is warmed
through. Serve immediately.

PER SERVING
carbs: 7 grams; Net Carbs: 3.5 grams;
fiber: 3.5 grams; protein: 9.5 grams; fat: 11.5 grams; calories: 166

PHASES 2–4

SOUPS

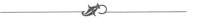

Cream of Watercress Soup
Avocado Soup
French Onion Soup Gratinée
Asparagus and Leek Soup
Roasted Pepper Soup
Cucumber Dill Soup
Mediterranean Vegetable Soup
Miso Soup
Turkey-Lemon Soup

CREAM OF WATERCRESS SOUP

The watercress is only slightly cooked, giving this soup a fresh, peppery flavor. It is ideal as a first course with Veal Saltimbocca (page 120).

(page 120)

PREP TIME: 20 MINUTES • COOK TIME: 20 MINUTES

4 SERVINGS

2 tablespoons butter

1 cup chopped onion

2 cups reduced-sodium chicken broth

1½ cups chopped cauliflower

4 bunches watercress, stems removed

⅔ cup heavy cream

salt and pepper to taste

nutmeg to taste

1. Heat the butter in a large saucepan over medium-high heat until the foam subsides. Add the onion and sauté for 5 minutes, stirring occasionally. Add the chicken broth and cauliflower and bring to a boil. Lower the heat, cover, and simmer for 10 minutes.

2. Turn off the heat and add the watercress. Cover and let stand for 5 minutes, stirring once.

3. Transfer the mixture to a food processor and add the cream, salt, pepper, and nutmeg, and purée for 1 minute, or until smooth. Serve warm, or refrigerate and serve chilled.

PER SERVING

carbs: 7.5 grams; Net Carbs: 5 grams;

fiber: 2.5 grams; protein: 5 grams; fat: 21.5 grams; calories: 232

PHASES 1–4

AVOCADO SOUP

$\mathcal{S}$imple and delicate, this creamy soup makes a sublime starter for Rack of Lamb with Brussels Sprouts (page 113).

PREP TIME: 15 MINUTES • COOK TIME: 10 MINUTES
4 SERVINGS

2 tablespoons butter
2 scallions (white part only), finely
    chopped
3 cups reduced-sodium chicken
    broth

2 Haas avocados, peeled, pitted,
    and drizzled with lemon juice
⅔ cup heavy cream
salt and pepper to taste

1. Heat the butter in a skillet over medium heat until the foam subsides. Add the scallions and cook, stirring occasionally, for 2 minutes, or until translucent. Add 2½ cups of the chicken broth, bring to a boil, then lower the heat and simmer for 3 minutes.

2. In a food processor, blend the avocados, cream, and remaining ½ cup broth until smooth.

3. Add the avocado mixture to the skillet and cook over medium heat, stirring occasionally, for 2 minutes, or until heated through. Season with salt and pepper, and serve.

PER SERVING
carbs: 8.5 grams; Net Carbs: 4 grams;
fiber: 4.5 grams; protein: 5 grams; fat: 36.5 grams; calories: 363

PHASES 1—4

FRENCH ONION SOUP GRATINÉE

This comforting soup was one of Dr. Atkins' all-time favorites. Serve it with Mixed Green Salad with Warm Bacon Dressing (page 44) for a satisfying light supper.

PREP TIME: 10 MINUTES • COOK TIME: 15 MINUTES
4 SERVINGS

2 tablespoons olive oil

2 medium onions, thinly sliced

two 14-ounce cans reduced-
    sodium chicken broth

¼ cup dry sherry

2 tablespoons Worcestershire sauce

1 cube beef bouillon

½ cup grated Parmesan cheese

salt and pepper to taste

¼ pound Swiss cheese, grated

1. Preheat the broiler. Heat the oil in a large saucepan over medium-low heat until hot but not smoking. Add the onions and cook, stirring occasionally, for 10 minutes, or until golden.

2. Raise the heat to medium-high and stir in the chicken broth, sherry, Worcestershire sauce, and bouillon cube. Bring to a boil, then lower the heat and simmer for 3 minutes. Add the Parmesan, salt, and pepper, and simmer for another 3 minutes.

3. Transfer the soup to 4 large flameproof serving bowls and top with the Swiss cheese. Broil for 1–2 minutes, until the cheese is melted and golden brown. Serve immediately.

PER SERVING
carbs: 9.5 grams; Net Carbs: 8.5 grams;
fiber: 1 gram; protein: 16.5 grams; fat: 19 grams; calories: 283

PHASES 2–4

ASPARAGUS AND LEEK SOUP

*H*ere's a simple soup in which the taste of the vegetables really comes through. Recipes often call for soups like this to be strained, but I prefer the earthy texture of this more rustic version.

PREP TIME: 15 MINUTES • COOK TIME: 15 MINUTES
6 SERVINGS

2 tablespoons butter

2 leeks (white part only), halved lengthwise, washed well, and chopped

1½ pounds asparagus, cut into ½-inch pieces

two 14-ounce cans reduced-sodium chicken broth

½ cup heavy cream

salt and pepper to taste

1. Heat the butter in a large saucepan over medium-high heat until the foam subsides. Add the leeks and sauté, stirring, for 2 minutes. Add the asparagus and sauté, stirring, for 1 minute. Add the chicken broth and bring the mixture to a boil. Lower the heat, cover, and simmer for 8–10 minutes, or until the asparagus is tender.

2. Transfer the mixture to a food processor. Add the cream, salt, and pepper. Purée for 1 minute, or until smooth. Serve immediately.

PER SERVING
carbs: 11 grams; Net Carbs: 8.5 grams;
fiber: 2.5 grams; protein: 6 grams; fat: 12.5 grams; calories: 171

PHASES 2—4

ROASTED PEPPER SOUP

*F*lavorful Parmesan cheese and sweet roasted peppers make this soup a treat for your taste buds.

PREP TIME: 20 MINUTES • COOK TIME: 15 MINUTES
4 SERVINGS

¼ cup olive oil

2 celery stalks, trimmed and
    chopped

⅔ cup chopped onion

2 cloves garlic, minced

4 yellow or red bell peppers,
    roasted, peeled, seeded, and
    chopped

3 cups reduced-sodium chicken
    broth

⅔ cup heavy cream

salt and pepper to taste

½ cup grated Parmesan cheese

1. Heat the oil in a skillet over medium heat until hot but not smoking. Add the celery, onion, and garlic, and cook, stirring occasionally, for about 5 minutes, or until the celery is soft. Add the peppers and chicken broth. Bring to a boil, then lower the heat and simmer for 3 minutes.

2. Transfer the mixture to a food processor. Add the cream, salt, and pepper. Process until smooth, about 45 seconds. Ladle the soup into 4 serving bowls and sprinkle Parmesan on top. Serve immediately.

PER SERVING
carbs: 14.5 grams; Net Carbs: 12.5 grams;
fiber: 2 grams; protein: 9 grams; fat: 32.5 grams; calories: 375

PHASES 3 AND 4

CUCUMBER DILL SOUP

During the warm-weather months, I like to keep a container of this refreshing soup in the refrigerator for a quick afternoon snack. Serve chilled with sour cream, if desired.

PREP TIME: 10 MINUTES • COOK TIME: 15 MINUTES
4 SERVINGS

2 tablespoons olive oil
⅔ cup chopped onion
2 large cucumbers, peeled, seeded, and cut crosswise into ½-inch slices

2 cups reduced-sodium chicken broth
2 tablespoons balsamic vinegar
2 tablespoons chopped fresh dill
salt and pepper to taste

1. Heat the oil in a large saucepan over medium-high heat until hot but not smoking. Add the onion and cook, stirring, for 2 minutes. Add the cucumber and chicken broth and bring to a boil. Lower the heat, cover, and simmer for 10 minutes. Stir in the vinegar, dill, salt, and pepper.

2. Transfer the mixture to a food processor and purée for 1 minute, or until smooth. Refrigerate for at least 1 hour before serving.

PER SERVING
carbs: 7.5 grams; Net Carbs: 6 grams;
fiber: 1.5 grams; protein: 2.5 grams; fat: 8 grams; calories: 107

PHASES 2–4

MEDITERRANEAN VEGETABLE SOUP

*T*his hearty and filling soup makes a lovely lunch when accompanied by a salad.

PREP TIME: 20 MINUTES • COOK TIME: 20 MINUTES
4 SERVINGS

½ tablespoon olive oil

½ cup chopped onion

1 clove garlic, minced

2 cups water

one 14-ounce can reduced-sodium chicken broth

½ cup chopped tomatoes in tomato juice

1 cup chopped kale

½ cup sliced mushrooms

½ cup sliced green beans

½ cup diced zucchini

½ cup diced yellow squash

1 tablespoon chopped fresh basil

2 tablespoons grated Parmesan cheese

1. Heat the olive oil in a heavy 2-quart saucepan over medium-low heat. Add the onion and cook, stirring occasionally, for 5 minutes, or until soft. Add the garlic and cook until fragrant. Stir in the water, broth, and tomatoes, and bring to a boil. Add the kale and bring the soup to a boil, then lower the heat, cover, and cook for 10 minutes.

2. Add the mushrooms, green beans, zucchini, and yellow squash. Bring to a boil, then reduce to medium and cook, uncovered, for 10 minutes.

3. Divide the soup among bowls and garnish with the basil and Parmesan.

PER SERVING
carbs: 7.5 grams; Net Carbs: 5.5 grams;
fiber: 2 grams; protein: 5 grams; fat: 3.5 grams; calories: 76

PHASES 1−4

MISO SOUP

*M*iso paste and bok choy are usually available in specialty- or natural-food stores. You may substitute napa cabbage if bok choy is unavailable. Edamame (young soy beans) are usually found in the freezer section.

PREP TIME: 15 MINUTES • COOK TIME: 8 MINUTES
4 SERVINGS

1 quart water

4 tablespoons miso paste

1½ cups thinly sliced bok choy

1 cup thinly sliced shiitake
    mushroom caps

½ cup edamame

1 cup diced firm tofu

½ scallion, thinly sliced

1. Heat the water in a large saucepan over medium-high heat and whisk in the miso paste. Bring to a boil. Add the bok choy and mushrooms and return to a boil. Reduce the heat and simmer for 3–4 minutes.

2. Add the edamame and tofu, return to a simmer, then remove from heat. Serve the soup immediately, garnished with the scallion.

PER SERVING
carbs: 14.5 grams; Net Carbs: 11.5 grams;
fiber: 3 grams; protein: 12 grams; fat: 6 grams; calories: 147

PHASES 1–4

TURKEY-LEMON SOUP

A small amount of lemon zest and a squeeze of juice add a bright flavor to this soup, which can be on the table in less than 20 minutes.

PREP TIME: 10 MINUTES • COOK TIME: 8 MINUTES

4 SERVINGS

1 tablespoon olive oil

1 scallion, finely chopped

two 14½-ounce cans reduced-
  sodium chicken broth

1 cup water

1¼ pounds turkey breast, cut into
  ½-inch cubes

½ teaspoon dried sage

½ teaspoon dried thyme

1 teaspoon grated lemon zest

1 tablespoon lemon juice

salt and pepper to taste

1. Heat the oil in a large saucepan over medium heat. Add the scallion and cook for 1 minute, until softened. Add the broth, water, turkey, sage, and thyme, and bring to a boil. Reduce the heat and simmer for 5 minutes, until the turkey is almost cooked through.

2. Add the lemon zest and juice. Cook for 2–3 minutes more. Add the salt and pepper.

PER SERVING

carbs: 3 grams; Net Carbs: 3 grams;
fiber: 0 grams; protein: 31 grams; fat: 16 grams; calories: 286

PHASES 1–4

SALADS

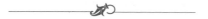

Greek Salad

Orange Daikon Salad

Red Cabbage Salad with Feta and Dill

Walnut Coleslaw

Fennel Salad with Parmesan

Celery Root Salad

Endive Salad with Walnuts and Roquefort

Mixed Green Salad with Warm Bacon Dressing

Shrimp Salad with Hearts of Palm

Crunchy Spinach Salad

GREEK SALAD

This snappy salad makes a delicious lunch or first course.

PREP TIME: 20 MINUTES

4 SERVINGS

2 tablespoons red wine vinegar

salt and pepper to taste

⅓ cup olive oil

2 medium tomatoes, cut into
    2-inch cubes

2 cucumbers, peeled, seeded, and
    thinly sliced

⅔ cup crumbled feta cheese

½ cup thinly sliced red onion

4 Kalamata olives, cut into slivers
    (1 tablespoon)

1. In a large serving bowl, whisk together the vinegar, salt, and pepper. Drizzle the oil in a steady stream and whisk until combined.

2. Add the tomatoes, cucumbers, feta, onion, and olives, and toss well. Serve immediately.

PER SERVING

carbs: 8 grams; Net Carbs: 6.5 grams;
fiber: 1.5 grams; protein: 5 grams; fat: 24 grams; calories: 256

PHASES 1–4

ORANGE DAIKON SALAD

If you can't find daikon—a mild radish—you can substitute jicama for an equally pleasing crunch. Jicama is a baseball-sized tuber with a slightly sweet flavor.

PREP TIME: 15 MINUTES

4 SERVINGS

—————————— ✑ ——————————

2 tablespoons red wine vinegar

2 teaspoons grated orange zest

salt to taste

¼ cup sunflower oil

about 2 pounds daikon radish or

    jicama, peeled and thinly sliced

    (4 cups)

1. In a large serving bowl, whisk together the vinegar, orange zest, and salt. Drizzle the oil in a steady stream and whisk until combined.

2. Add the daikon to the dressing and toss well. Serve immediately.

PER SERVING

carbs: 7 grams; Net Carbs: 4 grams;

fiber: 3 grams; protein: 2.5 grams; fat: 14 grams; calories: 156

PHASES 1–4

Red Cabbage Salad with Feta and Dill

A friend created this colorful salad for a potluck dinner, and it has been her most requested dish for informal get-togethers and picnics ever since.

PREP TIME: 20 MINUTES

4 SERVINGS

2 tablespoons lemon juice

2 cloves garlic, minced

salt and pepper to taste

½ cup olive oil

1 pound red cabbage, chopped
(about 3 cups)

1 cup crumbled feta cheese

⅓ cup chopped fresh dill

½ cup pine nuts, lightly toasted

1. In a large serving bowl, whisk together the lemon juice, garlic, salt, and pepper. Drizzle the oil in a steady stream and whisk until combined.

2. Add the cabbage, feta, dill, and pine nuts, and toss well. Serve immediately.

PER SERVING

carbs: 8.5 grams; Net Carbs: 6.5 grams;
fiber: 2 grams; protein: 7.5 grams; fat: 29.5 grams; calories: 313

PHASES 2−4

WALNUT COLESLAW

*C*runchy and fresh, this salad of sprouts and walnuts is a delicious twist on the more traditional recipe.

PREP TIME: 20 MINUTES
4 SERVINGS

½ cup mayonnaise

2 tablespoons Dijon mustard

2 teaspoons balsamic vinegar

salt and pepper to taste

1 cup chopped red cabbage

1 cup chopped celery

½ cup chopped walnuts

1. In a large serving bowl, whisk together the mayonnaise, mustard, vinegar, salt, and pepper.

2. Add the cabbage, celery, and walnuts, and mix well. Serve immediately.

PER SERVING
carbs: 6 grams; Net Carbs: 4 grams;
fiber: 2 grams; protein: 3.5 grams; fat: 32.5 grams; calories: 317

PHASES 2–4

FENNEL SALAD WITH PARMESAN

This is one of my favorite summer salads. The flavors are clean and fresh, and the Parmesan gives it just the right saltiness. For an elegant presentation, use a vegetable peeler to shave the Parmesan into paper-thin slices.

PREP TIME: 20 MINUTES

6 SERVINGS

2 tablespoons white wine vinegar

2 tablespoons chopped fresh dill

2 tablespoons chopped fresh
   flat-leaf parsley

salt and pepper to taste

⅓ cup olive oil

2 fennel bulbs (about 1½ pounds),
   halved lengthwise, cored, and
   very thinly sliced

18 shavings Parmesan cheese or
   ¼ cup grated Parmesan cheese

1. In a large serving bowl, whisk together the vinegar, dill, parsley, salt, and pepper. Drizzle the oil in a steady stream and whisk until combined.

2. Add the fennel and toss gently. Garnish with Parmesan and serve immediately.

PER SERVING

carbs: 13 grams; Net Carbs: 8.5 grams;

fiber: 4.5 grams; protein: 4.5 grams; fat: 13 grams; calories: 237

PHASES 2–4

CELERY ROOT SALAD

*C*elery root has a clean flavor and a crunchy texture. It's a seasonal vegetable, not available year-round, but an equal amount of chopped celery can be substituted. Serve this salad with Spiced Skirt Steak (page 130).

PREP TIME: 20 MINUTES

4 SERVINGS

¼ cup mayonnaise

4 teaspoons red wine vinegar

2 teaspoons Dijon mustard

salt and pepper to taste

1 pound celery root, peeled and
   coarsely chopped (about 2 cups)

2 tablespoons chopped fresh
   cilantro or parsley

1. In a large bowl, whisk together the mayonnaise, vinegar, mustard, salt, and pepper.

2. Add the celery root and mix well. Sprinkle with cilantro or parsley and serve immediately.

PER SERVING
carbs: 11.5 grams; Net Carbs: 9.5 grams;
fiber: 2 grams; protein: 2 grams; fat: 11.5 grams; calories: 151

PHASES 2–4

ENDIVE SALAD WITH
WALNUTS AND ROQUEFORT

The pretty presentation of this salad makes it ideal for a special-occasion meal. You can double or triple the recipe as needed.

PREP TIME: 20 MINUTES

4 SERVINGS

2 teaspoons fresh lemon juice

2 teaspoons fresh orange juice

2 teaspoons grated orange zest

salt and pepper to taste

⅔ cup crumbled Roquefort or other
    blue cheese

¼ cup olive oil

2 plump heads of endive, leaves
    separated, washed well, and
    spun dry

⅔ cup chopped walnuts, lightly
    toasted

1. In a small bowl, whisk together the lemon juice, orange juice, orange zest, salt, and pepper. Whisk in the Roquefort and oil (if the cheese clumps, mash it with a fork).

2. Arrange the endive leaves like the spokes of a wheel on a serving plate. Pour the Roquefort dressing over the endive and sprinkle the walnuts on top. Serve immediately.

PER SERVING
carbs: 12.5 grams; Net Carbs: 3 grams;
fiber: 9.5 grams; protein: 11.5 grams; fat: 34.5 grams; calories: 387

PHASES 2−4

MIXED GREEN SALAD WITH
WARM BACON DRESSING

*S*moky bacon and sweet sautéed leek combine in a flavor-packed salad dressing that blends beautifully with assorted greens.

PREP TIME: 15 MINUTES • COOK TIME: 10 MINUTES
4 SERVINGS

2 ounces slab bacon, cut into
    ½-inch cubes
1 leek (white part only), halved
    lengthwise, washed well, and
    thinly sliced
2 tablespoons olive oil

1 tablespoon red wine vinegar
8 cups torn assorted lettuce leaves
    (Boston, romaine, red leaf),
    washed and dried
salt and pepper to taste

1. In a medium skillet, cook the bacon over medium heat for 2–3 minutes, until golden. Add the leeks and cook for 4 minutes more, until the bacon is brown and the leeks are softened. Reduce the heat to low and add the oil and vinegar. Cook, stirring, for 30 seconds.

2. Place the lettuce leaves in a large bowl. Pour the warm dressing on top. Toss well, and season with salt and pepper. Serve immediately.

PER SERVING
carbs: 6 grams; Net Carbs: 4.5 grams;
fiber: 1.5 grams; protein: 3 grams; fat: 9 grams; calories: 116

PHASES 1–4

SHRIMP SALAD WITH HEARTS OF PALM

*H*earts of palm are available in jars or cans in most supermarkets. They resemble thick white asparagus stems and have a tart, clean flavor. This main-dish salad is fit for a special luncheon.

PREP TIME: 15 MINUTES
4 SERVINGS

½ cup bottled low carbohydrate
   Italian dressing
1 tablespoon lime juice
2 teaspoons lime zest
2 teaspoons chopped fresh cilantro
½ teaspoon ground cumin
1 avocado, peeled and thinly sliced

1 small head iceberg lettuce,
   chopped (about 8 cups)
1 pound medium shrimp, cooked,
   peeled, and deveined
four 4-inch pieces canned or jarred
   hearts of palm, patted dry and
   cut into ¼-inch rounds

1. In a small bowl, whisk together the dressing, lime juice, lime zest, cilantro, and cumin.

2. In another small bowl, gently toss the avocado slices with ¼ cup of the dressing mixture. Set aside.

3. Divide the lettuce among 4 plates. On each plate, arrange ¼ of the avocado slices and ¼ of the shrimp in concentric circles. Mound ¼ of the hearts of palm in the centers. Pour the remaining dressing over the salads.

PER SERVING
carbs: 13.5 grams; Net Carbs: 9 grams;
fiber: 4.5 grams; protein: 26.5 grams; fat: 24 grams; calories: 369

PHASES 2–4

CRUNCHY SPINACH SALAD

This salad can be finished at the table to add a little show to a dinner party. It also makes a great lunch with the addition of some cold roast turkey and ham.

PREP TIME: 25 MINUTES
4 SERVINGS

DRESSING

1 clove garlic, minced	2 tablespoons Dijon mustard
¾ teaspoon salt	¼ cup olive oil
¼ teaspoon freshly ground pepper	1 tablespoon balsamic vinegar

SALAD

4 cups washed, torn spinach	½ cup sliced cucumber
2 cups washed, torn radicchio	½ cup sliced white mushrooms
½ cup sliced celery	½ cup chopped red bell pepper
½ cup sliced radishes	⅓ cup crumbled blue cheese

1. Make the dressing: In a salad bowl, mix the garlic, salt, and pepper to make a paste. Let stand for 5 minutes. Add the mustard and slowly whisk in half of the olive oil. Whisk in the vinegar and then the remaining oil.

2. Make the salad: Add the spinach, radicchio, celery, radishes, cucumber, mushrooms, and red pepper to the salad bowl and toss well to coat thoroughly with the dressing.

3. Sprinkle the salad with blue cheese and serve immediately.

PER SERVING
carbs: 7 grams; Net Carbs: 5 grams;
fiber: 2 grams; protein: 5 grams; fat: 18 grams; calories: 200

PHASES 1–4

BREAKFASTS

Poached Eggs
Mustard Scrambled Eggs
Baked Eggs with Swiss Cheese and Cream
Ricotta and Leek Frittata
Smoked Salmon Frittata
Eggs Benedict with Spinach
Sunday Pancakes
Orange Waffles
Almond French Toast
Pecan-Maple Bread Pudding
Pumpkin Cranberry Muffins
Mixed Berry Muffins
Peach Breakfast Pudding

POACHED EGGS

*P*oaching *is a wonderful way to prepare eggs, and poached eggs are the basis of any number of classic dishes, such as Eggs Benedict. The addition of vinegar to the water helps the egg whites hold their shape.*

PREP TIME: 15 MINUTES • COOK TIME: 2–3 MINUTES
4 SERVINGS

2 tablespoons white vinegar
2 teaspoons salt

8 large eggs

1. In a large, deep skillet, add water until it is 1 inch deep. Bring to a boil. Add the vinegar and salt, and lower the heat so that the water just simmers.

2. Crack the eggs, one at a time, into a saucer or small bowl, being careful not to break the yolks. Slip them one at a time into the water. Poach the eggs over low heat for 2–3 minutes, until the whites are firm.

3. Remove the eggs with a slotted spoon. Serve immediately.

PER SERVING
carbs: 1 gram; Net Carbs: 1 gram;
fiber: 0 grams; protein: 12 grams; fat: 10 grams; calories: 150

PHASES 1–4

MUSTARD SCRAMBLED EGGS

*D*r. Atkins loved to make breakfast on weekends, and he often came up with unusual and tasty combinations. This was one of his favorites. Serve with bacon or sausage on the side.

PREP TIME: 5 MINUTES • COOK TIME: 5 MINUTES
4 SERVINGS

8 eggs

¼ cup sour cream

2 tablespoons hot water

1½ teaspoons dry mustard

¾ teaspoon dried oregano

4 tablespoons butter

salt and pepper to taste

1. Combine the eggs, sour cream, water, mustard, and oregano in a bowl and beat lightly.
2. Heat the butter in a skillet over medium heat until the foam subsides. Add the egg mixture and cook, stirring, for about 4 minutes, until the mixture becomes custardlike but not loose.
3. Season with salt and pepper, and serve immediately.

PER SERVING
carbs: 2 grams; Net Carbs: 2 grams;
fiber: 0 grams; protein: 13.5 grams; fat: 25.5 grams; calories: 295

PHASES 1–4

BAKED EGGS WITH
SWISS CHEESE AND CREAM

Baked eggs, or shirred eggs, make great individual meals. This recipe calls for 10-ounce ramekins, but if you have only smaller ones, use one egg instead of two in each ramekin.

PREP TIME: 20 MINUTES • COOK TIME: 15 MINUTES

4 SERVINGS

4 tablespoons butter, softened

8 eggs

1 cup grated Swiss cheese

1 cup heavy cream, heated

salt and pepper to taste

1. Preheat the oven to 350°F.

2. Butter four 10-ounce ramekins and break 2 eggs into each one. Cover each portion with ¼ cup cheese and ¼ cup warm cream, and season with salt and pepper.

3. Place the ramekins in a roasting pan filled with enough water to come halfway up the sides of the ramekins. Bake for 15 minutes, or until the cheese begins to brown. Serve immediately.

PER SERVING
carbs: 3.5 grams; Net Carbs: 3.5 grams;
fiber: 0 grams; protein: 21.5 grams; fat: 51.5 grams; calories: 563

PHASES 1–4

RICOTTA AND LEEK FRITTATA

*L*eeks become marvelously sweet when they are sautéed. Here, they give an extra measure of flavor to this frittata. Serve with a mixed green salad.

PREP TIME: 10 MINUTES • COOK TIME: 10 MINUTES
4 SERVINGS

2 tablespoons butter, divided
2 leeks (white part only), halved
   lengthwise, washed well, and
   cut into ½-inch pieces

8 eggs, lightly beaten
3 tablespoons whole-milk ricotta
   cheese
salt and pepper to taste

1. Preheat the broiler. Heat 1 tablespoon of butter in a large ovenproof skillet (preferably nonstick) over medium-high heat until the foam subsides. Add the leeks and sauté, stirring, for 3 minutes. Remove from the heat and let cool.

2. In a large bowl, combine the sautéed leeks, beaten eggs, ricotta, salt, and pepper. Mix well.

3. Heat the remaining 1 tablespoon of butter in the skillet over medium heat until the foam subsides. Add the egg mixture and cook, stirring, for about 1 minute, until the egg starts to form curds. Cook for another minute. The egg mixture should be set on the bottom and still a bit wet on top.

4. Place the skillet under the broiler for about 2 minutes, until the frittata turns golden brown. Using a spatula, carefully remove the frittata from the skillet. Cut into 4 wedges and serve immediately.

PER SERVING
carbs: 7.5 grams; Net Carbs: 6.5 grams;
fiber: 1 gram; protein: 14.5 grams; fat: 18 grams; calories: 253

PHASES 1–4

SMOKED SALMON FRITTATA

*E*ggs are not just for breakfast. This elegant frittata is also perfect for a late supper. For special occasions, top it with sour cream and caviar.

PREP TIME: 10 MINUTES • COOK TIME: 10 MINUTES
4 SERVINGS

---

8 eggs

2 ounces smoked salmon, chopped

2 tablespoons sour cream

1 tablespoon chopped fresh chives

salt and pepper to taste

2 tablespoons butter

1. Preheat the broiler. In a bowl, beat together the eggs, salmon, sour cream, chives, salt, and pepper.

2. Heat the butter in a large ovenproof skillet (preferably nonstick) over medium heat until the foam subsides. Pour in the egg mixture and cook, stirring, for about 1 minute, until the egg mixture is set on the bottom and still a bit wet on top.

3. Place the skillet under the broiler and broil for about 2 minutes, until the frittata turns golden brown. Using a spatula, carefully remove the frittata from the skillet. Cut into 4 wedges and serve immediately.

PER SERVING
carbs: 1.5 grams; Net Carbs: 1.5 grams;
fiber: 0 grams; protein: 15.5 grams; fat: 18.5 grams; calories: 238

PHASES 1–4

EGGS BENEDICT WITH SPINACH

*E*ggs Benedict and Eggs Florentine combine in this savory dish. Serve as a lunch or brunch entrée.

PREP TIME: 15 MINUTES • COOK TIME: 10 MINUTES
4 SERVINGS

8 pieces Canadian bacon

2 cups cooked frozen or fresh
   spinach

8 Poached Eggs (page 49)

½ cup Quick & Easy Hollandaise
   (page 160)

1 tablespoon chopped fresh flat-leaf
   parsley or dill (optional)

1. Heat a skillet over medium heat until hot but not smoking. Add the Canadian bacon and cook for about 2 minutes on each side, until lightly browned.

2. Divide the spinach among 4 plates. Top each serving with 2 pieces of bacon and 2 poached eggs. Spoon the Hollandaise over the eggs and sprinkle with the parsley or dill if desired. Serve immediately.

PER SERVING
carbs: 7.5 grams; Net Carbs: 4.5 grams;
fiber: 3 grams; protein: 28.5 grams; fat: 32.5 grams; calories: 433

PHASES 1–4

VARIATION: For a different taste, substitute 8 small, thin slices of smoked salmon for the Canadian bacon.

SUNDAY PANCAKES

$\mathcal{T}$his makes a special Sunday brunch: scrumptious pancakes topped with egg, sausage, and cheese.

PREP TIME: 20 MINUTES • COOK TIME: 10 MINUTES
4 SERVINGS (8 PANCAKES)

PANCAKES

1 cup Atkins Quick Quisine ™
   Pancake & Waffle Mix
4 eggs

2 tablespoons vegetable oil
⅔ cup water

TOPPING

6 breakfast sausage links, cut into
   ½-inch pieces
8 eggs
salt and pepper to taste

½ cup grated cheddar cheese
½ cup sliced scallions
¼ cup sour cream

1. Make the pancakes: Double the pancake mix package recipe (using 4 eggs, 2 tablespoons oil, and ⅔ cup water) to make 8 pancakes. Cook according to package directions, using a scant ⅓ cup batter for each pancake. Keep the pancakes warm.

2. Make the topping: Heat a skillet over medium heat and cook the sausage for 4 minutes, or until golden brown.

3. In a bowl, beat 8 eggs and season with salt and pepper. Add to the sausage and scramble to desired doneness.

4. To serve, place 1 pancake on each of 4 plates. Top with ¼ of the eggs and sausage. Sprinkle the cheese and half of the scallions over the eggs. Top with the remaining pancakes, 1 tablespoon of sour cream, and the remaining scallions. Serve immediately.

PER SERVING
carbs: 9.5 grams; Net Carbs: 6 grams;
fiber: 3.5 grams; protein: 40 grams; fat: 38 grams; calories: 537

PHASES 1–4

ORANGE WAFFLES

This batter thickens as it sits and may need a little added water to return it to a pourable consistency. Waffles may be frozen and reheated in the oven. If you want to lower the carb count on this recipe, simply omit the orange.

PREP TIME: 20 MINUTES • COOK TIME: 10 MINUTES
4 SERVINGS (8 WAFFLES)

1½ cups Atkins Quick Quisine™
  Bake Mix
6 tablespoons granular sugar
  substitute
1 tablespoon baking powder
1 tablespoon grated orange zest
½ teaspoon salt
2 cups water

3 eggs, beaten
4 tablespoons unsalted butter,
  melted and cooled
1 cup heavy cream
nonstick cooking spray
1 large navel orange, peel and all
  pith removed, chopped into
  small pieces (1⅓ cups)

1. Heat a waffle iron. Chill a mixing bowl in the refrigerator.

2. In another bowl, combine the bake mix, 3 tablespoons of the sugar substitute, baking powder, orange zest, and salt. Mix in the water, eggs, and butter.

3. In the chilled bowl, beat the cream with the remaining 3 tablespoons of sugar substitute until soft peaks form.

4. Lightly spray the waffle iron with cooking spray. Pour ½ cup batter in the center of the waffle iron and cook until the steam stops and the waffle is crisp; set aside. Repeat with the remaining batter.

5. To serve, place 2 waffles on each of 4 plates. Top each serving with ½ cup whipped cream and ⅓ cup chopped orange. Serve immediately.

PER SERVING
carbs: 20 grams; Net Carbs: 14 grams;
fiber: 6 grams; protein: 33.5 grams; fat: 40.5 grams; calories: 566

PHASES 3 AND 4

ALMOND FRENCH TOAST

*A*n almond-flavored cream cheese filling sandwiched between two slices of French toast makes this breakfast a special treat.

PREP TIME: 10 MINUTES • COOK TIME: 10 MINUTES
4 SERVINGS

---

4 ounces cream cheese, softened

1 tablespoon granular sugar
    substitute

¼ teaspoon almond extract

8 slices Atkins Bakery™ Ready-to-
    Eat Sliced White Bread

4 eggs, beaten

½ cup heavy cream

½ cup water

½ teaspoon salt

⅛ teaspoon grated nutmeg

4 tablespoons unsalted butter

1 cup Atkins Quick Quisine™
    Sugar Free Pancake Syrup

½ cup sliced blanched almonds,
    toasted

1. Heat a griddle or large skillet.

2. Using a rubber spatula, thoroughly mix the cream cheese, sugar substitute, and almond extract in a bowl.

3. Spread ¼ of the cream cheese mixture on each of 4 slices of bread. Top with the remaining 4 bread slices.

4. In another bowl, combine the eggs, cream, water, salt, and nutmeg. Dip the sandwiches in the egg batter.

5. Heat the butter on the griddle until foaming subsides. Add the French toast sandwiches, in batches if necessary, and cook for about 3 minutes on each side, until golden brown. Transfer the sandwiches to warmed plates and top each with ¼ cup syrup and 2 tablespoons almonds. Serve immediately.

PER SERVING
carbs: 20 grams; Net Carbs: 10 grams;
fiber: 10 grams; protein: 26.5 grams; fat: 50.5 grams; calories: 626

PHASES 3 AND 4

PECAN-MAPLE BREAD PUDDING

This homey breakfast takes less than an hour to prepare and is a delightful way to start the day. By making this pudding in a water bath you are guaranteed a moist final product.

PREP TIME: 20 MINUTES • COOK TIME: 30 MINUTES
4 SERVINGS

nonstick cooking spray
4 slices Atkins Bakery™ Ready-to-
  Eat Sliced White Bread,
  lightly toasted and cut into
  ½-inch cubes
½ cup chopped pecans, toasted
1 cup heavy cream

1 cup water
3 eggs
⅓ cup Atkins Quick Quisine™
  Sugar Free Pancake Syrup
3 tablespoons granular sugar
  substitute

1. Preheat the oven to 325°F. Lightly coat a 4-cup ovenproof baking dish with cooking spray. Layer the bread cubes and pecans in the baking dish and set aside.

2. In a bowl, whisk together the cream, water, eggs, syrup, and sugar substitute. Pour the mixture over the bread and allow to sit for 15 minutes.

3. Place the baking dish in a larger pan and place in the oven. Pour enough hot water in the pan to come halfway up the sides of the baking dish. Bake for 30 minutes, or until a knife inserted in the middle of the pudding comes out clean. Remove from the oven and allow to cool slightly before serving.

PER SERVING
carbs: 13.5 grams; Net Carbs: 7 grams;
fiber: 6.5 grams; protein: 20 grams; fat: 39.5 grams; calories: 461

PHASES 2–4

PUMPKIN CRANBERRY MUFFINS

*P*umpkin purée is low in carbs and high in fiber, and it adds moisture to these tasty little muffins. If you can't find fresh or frozen cranberries, either leave them out or use half of a chopped apple instead.

PREP TIME: 20 MINUTES • COOK TIME: 35 MINUTES
12 MUFFINS

nonstick cooking spray
1 cup Atkins Quick Quisine™
   Bake Mix
½ cup very finely ground walnuts
2 teaspoons ground cinnamon
2 teaspoons baking powder

1 cup granular sugar substitute
1 cup pumpkin purée
2 eggs
½ cup canola oil
½ cup fresh or frozen cranberries,
   chopped

1. Preheat the oven to 350°F. Lightly coat two 6-compartment muffin pans with cooking spray.

2. In a large bowl, whisk the bake mix, walnuts, cinnamon, and baking powder. In a medium bowl, whisk the sugar substitute, pumpkin purée, eggs, and canola oil until well blended.

3. Add the pumpkin mixture to the bake mix mixture and stir just until moistened. Fold in the cranberries. Divide the batter among the muffin compartments.

4. Bake for 35 minutes, or until a toothpick inserted in the center of a muffin comes out clean. Cool the muffins in the pans for 5 minutes; then turn onto a wire rack to cool completely.

PER MUFFIN
carbs: 7 grams; Net Carbs: 5 grams;
fiber: 2 grams; protein: 8 grams; fat: 12.5 grams; calories: 167

PHASES 2–4

MIXED BERRY MUFFINS

In this recipe, be sure to use unsweetened berries. A mere half cup goes a long way: These little muffins—best served warm—explode with berry flavor.

PREP TIME: 10 MINUTES • COOK TIME: 30 MINUTES

12 MUFFINS

1 cup Atkins Quick Quisine™
   Bake Mix
¼ cup granular sugar substitute
½ cup sour cream
2 tablespoons butter, melted and
   cooled

2 tablespoons heavy cream
2 tablespoons water
½ cup frozen mixed berries

1. Preheat the oven to 350°F. Line a 12-compartment muffin pan with baking cups.

2. In a bowl, mix together the bake mix and sugar substitute. In another bowl, whisk together the sour cream, butter, heavy cream, and water.

3. Add the sour cream mixture to the bake mix mixture and stir until well combined. Fold in the berries. Divide the batter among the muffin compartments.

4. Bake for 30 minutes, or until toothpick inserted in the center of a muffin has moist crumbs and the muffin tops are browned. Cool the muffins in the pan for 10 minutes, then remove to a wire rack to cool completely.

PER MUFFIN
carbs: 4 grams; Net Carbs: 2.5 grams;
fiber: 1.5 grams; protein: 6.5 grams; fat: 6 grams; calories: 93

PHASES 2–4

PEACH BREAKFAST PUDDING

*T*his recipe is based on a French custard dessert. It is not too sweet and is a wonderful treat any time of day. It comes together in 10 minutes and is then popped in the oven.

PREP TIME: 10 MINUTES • COOK TIME: 45 MINUTES
4 SERVINGS

4 tablespoons butter

4 tablespoons Atkins Quick
   Quisine™ Bake Mix, divided

2 tablespoons granular sugar
   substitute

pinch salt

⅔ cup heavy cream

⅓ cup water

3 eggs

½ teaspoon vanilla extract

1 large peach, finely chopped

1. Preheat the oven to 350°F. Melt the butter in a pie plate in the oven.

2. In a medium bowl, mix 3 tablespoons bake mix, sugar substitute, and salt.

3. In a small bowl, whisk the cream, water, eggs and vanilla. Pour the liquid mixture into the dry ingredients and mix until smooth.

4. Toss the peaches with remaining 1 tablespoon of bake mix. Gently fold the peaches into the batter. Pour the batter into the buttered pie plate. Bake for 45 minutes, or until golden and puffy. Serve immediately.

PER SERVING
carbs: 7.5 grams; Net Carbs: 6 grams;
fiber: 1.5 grams; protein: 7 grams; fat: 29 grams; calories: 316

PHASES 3 AND 4

SEAFOOD

Stir-Fried Shrimp with Ginger and Mushrooms

Shrimp Scampi

Tarragon Shrimp Salad

Red Snapper with Tomato and Olives

Sautéed Sole

Scallops with Thyme

Scallops Meunière

Oven-Poached Salmon with Dill and Wine

Tuna with Ginger and Soy Sauce

Peppers Stuffed with Walnut Tuna Salad

Hazelnut-and-Pepper-Crusted Swordfish

Squid with Basil and Lime

Sautéed Soft-Shell Crabs

Crab and Avocado Salad

Baked Cod with Garlic and Tomato

Salmon Cakes

STIR-FRIED SHRIMP WITH GINGER AND MUSHROOMS

A quick and easy stir-fry is a perfect weekday supper. In this recipe you can substitute an equal amount of sliced chicken breast for the shrimp.

PREP TIME: 15 MINUTES • COOK TIME: 5 MINUTES
4 SERVINGS

2 tablespoons canola oil

3 cloves garlic, minced

¾ tablespoon peeled and chopped
    fresh ginger

1 cup sliced mushrooms

1 cup chopped celery

2 tablespoons toasted sesame oil

1½ pounds large shrimp, shelled
    and deveined

3 tablespoons reduced-sodium soy
    sauce

¾ teaspoon dried red pepper flakes,
    or to taste

1. Heat the canola oil in a large, heavy skillet or a wok over medium-high heat until hot but not smoking. Add the garlic and ginger, and stir-fry for 30 seconds. Add the mushrooms, celery, and sesame oil and stir-fry for 30 seconds.

2. Add the shrimp, soy sauce, and red pepper flakes, and stir-fry until the shrimp are pink and just cooked through, for 3–4 minutes. Serve immediately.

PER SERVING
carbs: 5 grams; Net Carbs: 4 grams;
fiber: 1 gram; protein: 36 grams; fat: 17 grams; calories: 324

PHASES 1–4

SHRIMP SCAMPI

*L*emon, wine, and garlic do wonders for shrimp. This dish is very easy to make and always a hit. You can easily double the recipe to serve guests.

PREP TIME: 15 MINUTES • COOK TIME: 10 MINUTES
4 SERVINGS

4 tablespoons butter

¼ cup olive oil

1 cup dry white wine

6 large cloves garlic, minced

¼ cup fresh lemon juice

pinch of dried red pepper flakes

salt and pepper to taste

2 pounds large shrimp, shelled and
    deveined

⅓ cup chopped fresh flat-leaf
    parsley

1. Heat the butter and oil in a heavy skillet over medium heat until the foam subsides. Add the wine, garlic, lemon juice, red pepper flakes, salt, and pepper. Bring to a boil, lower the heat, and simmer for 3 minutes.

2. Add the shrimp to the skillet and cook, stirring frequently, until the shrimp are pink, 3–5 minutes. Add the parsley 1 minute before the shrimp are done.

3. Place the shrimp on a serving plate and pour the sauce from the skillet over them. Serve immediately.

PER SERVING
carbs: 6.5 grams; Net Carbs: 6 grams;
fiber: 0.5 gram; protein: 47 grams; fat: 29 grams; calories: 517

PHASES 1–4

TARRAGON SHRIMP SALAD

*C*ool and refreshing, this tarragon-infused shrimp salad is a perfect light luncheon meal. Serve it on a bed of crisp mixed greens.

PREP TIME: 15 MINUTES
4 SERVINGS

¼ cup mayonnaise

2 tablespoons Dijon mustard

2 tablespoons drained nonpareil
capers

1 tablespoon chopped fresh flat-leaf
parsley

2 teaspoons chopped fresh tarragon
or 1 teaspoon dried tarragon

¾ teaspoon Anchovy Paste
(page 159), or 2 oil-packed
anchovy fillets, mashed

salt and pepper to taste

1½ pounds medium shrimp,
cooked, shelled, and deveined

In a large serving bowl, whisk together the mayonnaise, mustard, capers, parsley, tarragon, Anchovy Paste, salt, and pepper. Add the shrimp and toss the salad well. Serve immediately.

PER SERVING
carbs: 3 grams; Net Carbs: 3 grams;
fiber: 0 grams; protein: 35.5 grams; fat: 15 grams; calories: 293

PHASES 1–4

RED SNAPPER WITH
TOMATO AND OLIVES

he lusty flavor of classic Italian puttanesca sauce—tomatoes, capers, black olives—has a wonderful affinity for firm-fleshed red snapper. Serve with Wax Beans with Garlic-Tarragon Vinaigrette (page 133).

PREP TIME: 15 MINUTES • COOK TIME: 15 MINUTES
4–6 SERVINGS

2 tablespoons olive oil

1 small onion, chopped

1½ cloves garlic, minced

10 black Greek olives, pitted and
    chopped

1½ cups chopped tomatoes

½ cup dry red wine

3 tablespoons drained nonpareil
    capers

pinch of dried red pepper flakes
    (optional)

4 tablespoons butter

3 pounds red snapper fillets

1. Heat the oil in a large skillet over medium heat until hot but not smoking. Add the onion, garlic, and olives, and cook, stirring occasionally, for 3 minutes, or until the onion is transparent. Add the tomatoes, wine, capers, and red pepper flakes, if using. Bring to a boil, lower the heat, and simmer for 5 minutes.

2. Meanwhile, heat 2 tablespoons of the butter in another large skillet over medium heat until the foam subsides. Add half of the snapper fillets and cook for 2 minutes on each side, or until lightly browned. Transfer the snapper to a plate. Repeat with the remaining butter and snapper fillets.

3. Place all of the cooked snapper on top of the tomato mixture in the skillet, cover, and cook over medium heat for 3 minutes, or until the snapper just flakes. Serve immediately.

PER SERVING
carbs: 4.5 grams; Net Carbs: 3.5 grams;
fiber: 1 gram; protein: 32.5 grams; fat: 15.5 grams; calories: 299

PHASES 1–4

SAUTÉED SOLE

This crispy sole is especially good when served with Caper Tartar Sauce (page 157).

PREP TIME: 10 MINUTES • COOK TIME: 10 MINUTES

4 SERVINGS

2½ pounds sole fillets

salt and pepper to taste

2 eggs, lightly beaten

1 cup Atkins Quick Quisine™
   Bake Mix

4 tablespoons butter

¼ cup olive oil

1. Season the sole fillets with salt and pepper. Dip the fillets in the egg and dredge in the bake mix, shaking off any excess.

2. Heat 2 tablespoons each of the butter and oil in a large skillet over medium-high heat until the foam subsides. Add half the sole fillets (do not crowd) and cook for 2 minutes on each side. Drain the fillets on paper towels.

3. Wipe out the skillet. Repeat with the remaining butter, oil, and sole fillets. Serve immediately.

PER SERVING
carbs: 6 grams; Net Carbs: 3 grams;
fiber: 3 grams; protein: 85 grams; fat: 33.5 grams; calories: 679

PHASES 1−4

Scallops with Thyme

he rich, succulent flavor of scallops is complemented here by the tangy lemon and fresh thyme.

PREP TIME: 15 MINUTES • COOK TIME: 5 MINUTES
4 SERVINGS

2½ teaspoons salt

1½ teaspoons cayenne pepper

2 pounds sea scallops, rinsed and patted dry

5 tablespoons butter

3 cloves garlic, minced

3 scallions (white part only), chopped

1½ tablespoons fresh thyme or 2 teaspoons crumbled dried thyme

2 tablespoons fresh lemon juice

1. Combine the salt and cayenne in a small bowl. Sprinkle the mixture all over the scallops.

2. Heat the butter in a large, heavy skillet or a wok over medium-high heat until it bubbles and begins to brown. Add the garlic and scallions, and cook, stirring, for 30 seconds. Add the scallops and thyme, and cook, turning the scallops, for about 4 minutes, until they are lightly browned.

3. Drizzle with the lemon juice and serve immediately.

PER SERVING
carbs: 7.5 grams; Net Carbs: 7 grams;
fiber: 0.5 gram; protein: 38.5 grams; fat: 16 grams; calories: 336

PHASES 1–4

SCALLOPS MEUNIÈRE

𝒻or scallops that will brown well, dry them thoroughly on paper towels. Also, purchase ivory- or cream-colored scallops instead of very white ones, which may have been soaked to increase their weight.

PREP TIME: 15 MINUTES • COOK TIME: 10 MINUTES
4 SERVINGS

───────────────── ✍ ─────────────────

2 tablespoons olive oil

2 pounds sea scallops, ligaments
    removed, rinsed

salt and pepper to taste

4 tablespoons unsalted butter

2 tablespoons fresh lemon juice

2 tablespoons dry white wine

2 tablespoons chopped fresh parsley

1. Heat the olive oil in a large nonstick or well-seasoned skillet over medium-high heat until hot but not smoking. Pat the scallops dry and season with salt and pepper. Add the scallops to the skillet, in batches if necessary, and cook for 2 minutes on each side, until golden brown. Transfer the scallops to a dish and keep warm. Pour off the oil from the pan and discard.

2. Add the butter to the pan and cook until the foaming subsides and the butter begins to brown. Stir in the lemon juice, wine, and parsley, shaking the pan to emulsify the sauce. Season with additional salt and pepper, if desired. Pour the sauce over the scallops and serve immediately.

PER SERVING
carbs: 6 grams; Net Carbs: 6 grams;
fiber: 0 grams; protein: 38 grams; fat: 20 grams; calories: 368

─────────────────────────────

PHASES 1−4

OVEN-POACHED SALMON
WITH DILL AND WINE

*F*resh salmon has a very delicate flavor, and oven-poaching keeps it moist and tasty. Serve the salmon warm with lemon wedges or chilled with Cucumber-Dill Sauce, Creamy Celery Sauce, or Horseradish Cream (pages 151, 152, and 153).

PREP TIME: 10 MINUTES • COOK TIME: 20 MINUTES
4 SERVINGS

one 1½-pound salmon steak (about 1 inch thick)
salt and pepper to taste
3 tablespoons chopped fresh dill

3 tablespoons fresh lemon or lime juice
3 tablespoons dry white wine
1 bay leaf

1. Preheat the oven to 375°F. Place the salmon steak on two layers of aluminum foil, twice as big as the salmon. Season with salt and pepper. Bring up the foil on all sides and carefully add the dill, lemon juice, wine, and bay leaf. Fold all sides of the foil together, creating a tent over the salmon, and crimp the edges of the foil to seal. Place the salmon tent on a baking sheet and bake for 20 minutes.

2. Carefully unwrap the top of the foil (the steam will be very hot). Gently transfer the salmon to a serving plate, discard the bay leaf, and pour any accumulated liquid in the foil pouch over the fish. Serve immediately.

PER SERVING
carbs: 1.5 grams; Net Carbs: 1.5 grams;
fiber: 0 grams; protein: 45 grams; fat: 24.5 grams; calories: 429

PHASES 1−4

TUNA WITH GINGER AND SOY SAUCE

The Asian flavors of fresh ginger and soy sauce make this tuna fragrant and delicious. If you do not have a grill, you can pan-sear the tuna over medium-high heat for 4 minutes on each side.

PREP TIME: 20 MINUTES • COOK TIME: 10 MINUTES
4 SERVINGS

---

4 tuna steaks, about 2 inches thick
   (1½ pounds total)
⅔ cup canola oil
⅔ cup rice wine vinegar

⅓ cup soy sauce
2 tablespoons chopped fresh ginger
4 teaspoons toasted sesame seeds
⅓ cup heavy cream

1. Preheat a grill.

2. Place the tuna in a shallow nonreactive dish. In a bowl, whisk together the oil, vinegar, soy sauce, and ginger. Pour the mixture over the tuna, cover, and refrigerate, turning it once, for 15 minutes. Remove the tuna from the marinade, pat it dry, and sprinkle with the sesame seeds. Grill for 4 minutes on each side.

3. While the tuna is grilling, pour the marinade into a skillet and bring to a boil. Cook for 5 minutes. Add the cream and simmer for 1 minute (do not let it boil).

4. Transfer the tuna to plates and pour the sauce on top. Serve immediately.

PER SERVING
carbs: 2.5 grams; Net Carbs: 2 grams;
fiber: 0.5 gram; protein: 42 grams; fat: 20 grams; calories: 363

PHASES 2–4

PEPPERS STUFFED WITH
WALNUT TUNA SALAD

*Y*ou'll never miss the bread with this zesty tuna salad. For a heartier winter lunch, grate cheese over the top and bake for a few minutes—it makes a terrific tuna melt.

PREP TIME: 15 MINUTES
4 SERVINGS

½ cup chopped walnuts

½ cup chopped scallions

¼ cup olive oil

¼ cup mayonnaise

2 tablespoons lemon juice

1 teaspoon Dijon mustard

½ teaspoon freshly ground pepper

salt to taste

two 6-ounce cans chunk white
   tuna, drained

2 bell peppers, stemmed, halved
   crosswise, and seeded

2 tablespoons chopped fresh parsley

4 thin lemon slices for garnish
   (optional)

1. Combine the walnuts, scallions, oil, mayonnaise, lemon juice, mustard, pepper, and salt in a bowl and mix well. Using a fork, gently stir in the tuna.

2. Fill each bell pepper half with one-fourth of the tuna mixture. Sprinkle with parsley and garnish with lemon slices if desired. Serve immediately.

PER SERVING

carbs: 9 grams; Net Carbs: 6.5 grams;
fiber: 2.5 grams; protein: 26 grams; fat: 30 grams; calories: 401

PHASES 2−4

HAZELNUT-AND-
PEPPER-CRUSTED SWORDFISH

*M*eaty and rich, swordfish steaks are perfect carriers for this aromatic crust.

PREP TIME: 15 MINUTES • COOK TIME: 10 MINUTES
4 SERVINGS

⅓ cup ground hazelnuts (or
   pistachios)
¼ cup coarsely ground fresh black
   pepper
2 tablespoons coarsely ground
   coriander

salt to taste
4 swordfish steaks (1½ pounds
   total)
4 tablespoons butter, softened
¼ cup lime juice

1. Preheat the broiler. In a small bowl, combine the hazelnuts, pepper, coriander, and salt. Rub the swordfish all over with the softened butter and pat on the nut-herb mixture.

2. Place the fish in the broiler pan without a rack. Pour the lime juice in the pan. Broil the swordfish for 8 minutes, turning once, until opaque throughout. Serve immediately.

PER SERVING
carbs: 9 grams; Net Carbs: 5 grams;
fiber: 4 grams; protein: 25.5 grams; fat: 22.5 grams; calories: 331

PHASES 2–4

SQUID WITH BASIL AND LIME

*S*weet basil blends beautifully with the mild, almost nutty flavor of squid. Squid freezes well, so if you don't have access to fresh squid, the frozen product is fine.

PREP TIME: 25 MINUTES • MARINATE TIME: 1 HOUR
COOK TIME: 5 TO 10 MINUTES
4 SERVINGS

2 pounds cleaned squid, bodies cut
  into ½-inch rings and tentacles
  halved
¼ cup plus 1–2 tablespoons
  olive oil, divided

juice of 2 limes
1 large clove garlic, minced
½ teaspoon hot pepper sauce
1 cup chopped fresh basil

1. Combine the squid, ¼ cup of the olive oil, lime juice, garlic, and hot pepper sauce in a bowl and mix well. Cover and marinate in the refrigerator for 1 hour.

2. Add 1 tablespoon of olive oil to a wok or heavy skillet. Heat at medium-high heat until the oil shimmers. Remove the squid from the marinade, pat dry, and add to the wok (you can cook the squid in two batches, adding more oil if needed). Cook, stirring frequently, for about 4 minutes, until the squid is opaque and tender.

3. Garnish with basil and serve immediately.

PER SERVING
carbs: 9.5 grams; Net Carbs: 9 grams;
fiber: 0.5 gram; protein: 35.5 grams; fat: 23.5 grams; calories: 398

PHASES 2–4

SAUTÉED SOFT-SHELL CRABS

*C*rispy and flavorful, soft-shell crabs are wonderful with a drizzling of lemon or with Caper Tartar Sauce (page 157).

PREP TIME: 10 MINUTES • COOK TIME: 10 MINUTES
4 SERVINGS

⅓ cup Atkins Quick Quisine™
   Bake Mix or soy flour
2 tablespoons ground hazelnuts or
   almonds
salt and pepper to taste

8 soft-shell crabs, washed and
   patted dry
2 tablespoons butter
2 tablespoons olive oil

1. Combine the bake mix, hazelnuts, salt, and pepper. Dredge the crabs in the flour mixture, shaking off any excess.

2. Heat the butter and oil in a heavy skillet over medium heat until hot but not smoking. Add the crabs, in batches if necessary, and cook for 4 to 5 minutes on each side. Drain on paper towels and serve immediately.

PER SERVING
carbs: 2 grams; Net Carbs: 1.5 grams;
fiber: 0.5 gram; protein: 13.5 grams; fat: 16 grams; calories: 206

PHASES 2–4

CRAB AND AVOCADO SALAD

The combination of earthy cumin and rich avocado makes this crab salad the perfect light lunch.

PREP TIME: 15 MINUTES
4 SERVINGS

¼ cup chopped celery

¼ cup chopped red bell pepper

¼ cup mayonnaise

¼ cup lemon juice

2 tablespoons drained capers

1 teaspoon cumin

salt and pepper to taste

8 ounces cooked crabmeat

2 medium Haas avocadoes, cubed

2 bunches watercress, stems
    removed

1. Combine the celery, bell pepper, mayonnaise, lemon juice, capers, cumin, salt, and pepper, and mix well. Gently mix in the crab and avocado.

2. Divide the watercress among 4 plates, top with the crab salad, and serve immediately.

PER SERVING
carbs: 10 grams; Net Carbs: 4 grams;
fiber: 6 grams; protein: 15 grams; fat: 27.5 grams; calories: 330

PHASES 1−4

BAKED COD WITH GARLIC AND TOMATO

This dish can be prepped in advance and kept wrapped in the refrigerator, making it ideal for a party. Just pop it in the oven when your guests arrive. Serve on a large platter with a few sprigs of parsley for an attractive presentation.

PREP TIME: 10 MINUTES • COOK TIME: 20 MINUTES
4 SERVINGS

4 tablespoons butter, softened and divided

1 large clove garlic, minced

four 8-ounce cod fillets

1 large tomato (about 8 ounces), sliced as thin as possible

2 tablespoons dry white wine

½ slice Atkins Bakery™ Ready-to-Eat Sliced White Bread, made into bread crumbs

1. Cook 1 tablespoon of the butter with the garlic in a small microwave-safe cup for 30 seconds, until the garlic begins to color. Mix garlic butter into remaining butter until incorporated. Preheat the oven to 400°F.

2. Spread both sides of the fillets with ⅔ of the garlic butter and place the fish in a nonreactive baking dish. Top each fillet with 2 to 3 tomato slices, overlapping slightly. Spread the remaining garlic butter over the tomato slices. Pour the wine into the baking dish.

3. Bake for 10 minutes. Remove the pan from the oven and baste the fish with the accumulated juices. Sprinkle each fillet with 1 tablespoon bread crumbs. Return the pan to the oven and bake the fish for another 10 minutes, until the crumbs are golden brown.

4. Transfer the fish to a serving platter, spoon the pan juices around the fish, and serve immediately.

PER SERVING
carbs: 4.5 grams; Net Carbs: 3.5 grams;
fiber: 1 gram; protein: 26 grams; fat: 19.5 grams; calories: 305

PHASES 1−4

SALMON CAKES

The salmon mixture can also be made into smaller cakes and served as finger food at a party.

PREP TIME: 15 MINUTES • COOK TIME: 25 MINUTES
4 SERVINGS (8 CAKES)

3 slices Atkins Bakery™ Ready-to-
    Eat Sliced White Bread
¼ cup olive oil
1½ cups chopped celery
¾ cup chopped onion
1 teaspoon salt
¾ teaspoon Old Bay® Seasoning

½ cup mayonnaise
2 tablespoons chopped cilantro
¾ teaspoon Worcestershire sauce
1½ pounds cooked and flaked
    salmon
Caper Tartar Sauce (page 157)
lemon wedges

1. Tear bread into pieces and place in a food processor. Pulse until crumbs form.

2. Heat 2 tablespoons of olive oil in a skillet over medium heat. Add the celery and onions, and cook, stirring occasionally, about 10 minutes, until soft but not brown. Stir in the salt and Old Bay Seasoning, and cook for 30 seconds. Remove from the heat and let cool.

3. When the vegetables are cool, mix with the mayonnaise, cilantro, and Worcestershire sauce in a bowl. Gently stir in the salmon and ¾ cup of bread crumbs. Form the mixture into 8 cakes. Dip the cakes into the remaining bread crumbs and pat gently to coat (the cakes should be moist enough for crumbs to stick).

4. Heat the remaining 2 tablespoons of olive oil in a large, heavy skillet over medium-high heat until hot but not smoking. Add the salmon cakes, in two batches if necessary, and cook for about 3 minutes on each side, until golden brown. Drain the cakes on paper towels.

5. Serve immediately with tartar sauce and lemon wedges.

PER SERVING
*carbs: 10.5 grams; Net Carbs: 6 grams;
fiber: 4.5 grams; protein: 25 grams; fat: 47.5 grams; calories: 566*

PHASES 1–4

POULTRY

Chicken Cordon Bleu

Quick-Grilled Chicken Caesar Salad

Cornish Hens with Apricot-Wine Sauce

Chicken with Lemon and Capers

"Breaded" Chicken Cutlets

Curry Chicken Salad with Cucumbers

Chicken Salad with Fennel and Pesto

Chicken Coconut Satay with Cilantro

Chicken with Cucumbers

Chicken Paprika

Chicken with Indian Spices

Creamed Chicken with Mushrooms

Tomatillo Chicken

Breast of Duck with Red Wine Sauce

CHICKEN CORDON BLEU

This delicious French classic is wonderful served with mushrooms sautéed in butter.

PREP TIME: 20 MINUTES • COOK TIME: 10 MINUTES

4 SERVINGS

½ cup Atkins Quick Quisine™
   Bake Mix or soy flour
salt and pepper to taste
2 eggs, lightly beaten
2 whole skinless, boneless chicken
   breasts, cut in half

4 thin slices Swiss cheese
4 thin slices boiled or baked ham
2 tablespoons olive oil

1. On a plate, mix the bake mix, salt, and pepper. Put the eggs on another plate.

2. Pound the chicken breasts until they are very thin, about ⅛ inch thick. Place 1 slice of Swiss cheese and 1 slice of ham on each chicken piece. Fold the chicken in half, creating a "sandwich." Dip the chicken in the eggs and then dredge in the bake mix, shaking off any excess.

3. Heat the oil in a skillet over medium-high heat until hot but not smoking. Cook the chicken for 4 or 5 minutes on each side, or until golden brown and cooked through. Serve immediately.

PER SERVING
carbs: 3.5 grams; Net Carbs: 2 grams;
fiber: 1.5 grams; protein: 32 grams; fat: 16.5 grams; calories: 290

PHASES 1−4

QUICK-GRILLED
CHICKEN CAESAR SALAD

To make this even faster, prepare the dressing and croutons the day before.

PREP TIME: 20 MINUTES • MARINATE TIME: 20 MINUTES
COOK TIME: 10 MINUTES
4 SERVINGS

3½ tablespoons extra-virgin
    olive oil

1 tablespoon fresh lemon juice

salt and pepper to taste

4 skinless, boneless chicken breast
    halves, slightly flattened (about
    6–7 ounces each)

2 slices Atkins Bakery™ Ready-to-
    Eat Sliced White Bread, cut
    into ½-inch cubes

1 recipe Caesar Salad Dressing
    (page 168)

10 cups torn romaine lettuce leaves

½ cup grated Parmesan cheese

1. In a large dish, whisk 3 tablespoons of the oil with the lemon juice, salt, and pepper. Add the chicken and turn to coat well. Cover and refrigerate for at least 20 minutes and up to 1 hour.

2. Heat the remaining ½ tablespoon of oil in a small skillet. Add the bread cubes, stirring often, until golden brown. Season the croutons with salt and pepper, and drain on a paper towel.

3. Preheat the grill or broiler. Remove the chicken from the marinade and pat dry. Grill or broil the chicken for 4–5 minutes on each side, until the juices run clear when the chicken is pierced with a knife. Transfer the chicken to a dish and keep warm.

4. Place the Caesar dressing in a large salad bowl, add lettuce, and toss well. Add the croutons and Parmesan and toss again lightly. Divide the salad evenly among 4 plates.

5. Slice each chicken breast in 5 pieces and place on the salad. Serve immediately.

PER SERVING
carbs: 9.5 grams; Net Carbs: 5 grams;
fiber: 4.5 grams; protein: 53.5 grams; fat: 40 grams; calories: 612

PHASES 1–4

CORNISH HENS WITH APRICOT-WINE SAUCE

s a special-occasion dish, these succulent game hens can't be beat.

PREP TIME: 20 MINUTES • COOK TIME: 15 MINUTES
4 SERVINGS

2 tablespoons butter

4 small Cornish hens, quartered
   (about 1 pound each)

⅔ cup reduced-sodium chicken
   broth

½ cup dry white wine

¼ cup sugar-free apricot jam

2 tablespoons fresh lime juice

2 teaspoons grated lime zest

salt and pepper to taste

1. Heat the butter in a large, heavy casserole or Dutch oven over medium-high heat until the foam subsides. Add the hens and cook, turning once, for 5 minutes on each side.

2. Add the chicken broth, wine, jam, lime juice, lime zest, salt, and pepper to the casserole, and bring to a boil. Partially cover, reduce the heat to medium, and cook for 15 minutes, or until the hens are cooked through. Serve immediately.

PER SERVING
carbs: 2 grams; Net Carbs: 2 grams;
fiber: 0 grams; protein: 69 grams; fat: 61.5 grams; calories: 883

PHASES 2–4

CHICKEN WITH LEMON AND CAPERS

*T*angy *capers are a natural partner for chicken. In this dish, the capers and lemon juice are mellowed when butter is whisked into the liquid, creating a rich sauce.*

PREP TIME: 10 MINUTES • COOK TIME: 15 MINUTES
4 SERVINGS

2 tablespoons olive oil

1½ pounds chicken cutlets

⅔ cup white wine

2 tablespoons fresh lemon juice

2 tablespoons drained capers

2 teaspoons lemon zest

3 tablespoons chilled butter,
    cut into pieces

1. Heat the oil in a large, heavy skillet over medium heat until hot but not smoking. Add the chicken and cook, turning once, for 3–4 minutes on each side, or until browned. Transfer the chicken to a plate and keep warm.

2. Add the wine, lemon juice, capers, and lemon zest to the skillet and bring to a boil, stirring and scraping up any browned bits from the bottom of the pan. Simmer for 2 minutes. Whisk in the butter, a piece at a time, and cook over low heat for 1 minute. Return the chicken to the pan to heat through.

3. Transfer the chicken to a serving platter. Pour the sauce over the chicken and serve immediately.

PER SERVING
carbs: 1.5 grams; Net Carbs: 1 gram;
fiber: 0.5 gram; protein: 40 grams; fat: 18 grams; calories: 353

PHASES 1–4

"BREADED" CHICKEN CUTLETS

*C*hicken cutlets are a quick and easy staple of home cooking. Serve this version in the traditional manner with a drizzling of lemon juice.

PREP TIME: 15 MINUTES • COOK TIME: 20 MINUTES
4 SERVINGS

1 egg, lightly beaten

¼ cup Atkins Quick Quisine™
   Bake Mix

¼ cup ground almonds

1½ pounds chicken cutlets

2 tablespoons olive or canola oil

2 tablespoons butter

1 tablespoon chopped fresh parsley
   for garnish

1. Put the egg on a large plate. Stir together the bake mix and almonds on a second plate. Dip each chicken cutlet into the egg and then into the breading, making sure the chicken is thoroughly coated. Shake off any excess.

2. Heat 1 tablespoon each of oil and butter in a large, heavy skillet over medium heat until hot but not smoking. Add half the chicken cutlets and cook until golden brown and cooked through, about 4 minutes per side. Transfer to a plate and keep warm. Repeat with the remaining oil, butter, and chicken, wiping out the pan if necessary.

3. Transfer the chicken cutlets to a platter, sprinkle with parsley, and serve immediately.

PER SERVING
carbs: 3 grams; Net Carbs: 1.5 grams;
fiber: 1.5 grams; protein: 43 grams; fat: 33 grams; calories: 485

PHASES 2–4

CURRY CHICKEN SALAD
WITH CUCUMBERS

The sweet and spicy flavor of curry powder contrasts with the coolness of cucumber in this aromatic salad. A touch of cinnamon adds a hint of intrigue.

PREP TIME: 20 MINUTES

4 SERVINGS

½ cup mayonnaise

1 scallion, finely chopped

1 tablespoon chopped fresh flat-leaf
   parsley

1½ teaspoons curry powder

1 teaspoon cider vinegar

¼ teaspoon cinnamon

salt and pepper to taste

3 cups cubed cooked chicken

⅓ cup chopped celery

½ cup peeled, seeded, and chopped
   cucumber

1. Whisk together the mayonnaise, scallion, parsley, curry powder, vinegar, cinnamon, salt, and pepper in a large serving bowl.

2. Add the chicken, celery, and cucumber, and toss well to combine. Serve immediately, or refrigerate, covered, for up to 1 day.

PER SERVING

carbs: 2 grams; Net Carbs: 1.5 grams;
fiber: 0.5 gram; protein: 30 grams; fat: 29 grams; calories: 392

PHASES 1–4

CHICKEN SALAD WITH
FENNEL AND PESTO

*B*asil pesto creates a delicious coating for this chicken salad punctuated by the licorice flavor of the fennel.

PREP TIME: 20 MINUTES • COOK TIME: ABOUT 5 MINUTES
4 SERVINGS

2 tablespoons butter

1½ pounds chicken cutlets, cut
   into 1-inch strips

2 tablespoons lemon juice

6 tablespoons Basil Pesto
   (page 161), divided

1 medium fennel bulb, halved,
   cored, and thinly sliced

1 cup chopped red bell pepper

salt and pepper to taste

1. Heat the butter in a skillet over medium-high heat until the foam subsides. Add the chicken, drizzle with the lemon juice, and cook, turning frequently, until golden, about 5 minutes. Stir in 4 tablespoons of the pesto, coating the chicken well.

2. Transfer the chicken to a large serving bowl. Add the fennel, bell pepper, remaining 2 tablespoons of pesto, salt, and pepper. Toss well. Serve immediately or refrigerate, covered, for up to 1 day.

PER SERVING
carbs: 9 grams; Net Carbs: 6 grams;
fiber: 3 grams; protein: 40 grams; fat: 20.5 grams; calories: 381

PHASES 2–4

CHICKEN COCONUT SATAY
WITH CILANTRO

he coconut milk marinade makes this chicken satay tender and juicy. This dish can also be prepared without the skewers. Peanut Dipping Sauce (page 156) is the traditional accompaniment.

PREP TIME: 30 MINUTES • COOK TIME: 7 MINUTES
4 SERVINGS

one 14-ounce can unsweetened
   coconut milk
⅓ cup chopped fresh cilantro
2 tablespoons lime juice
1 teaspoon chopped fresh jalapeño
   chili

1 small clove garlic, minced
salt and pepper to taste
1½ pounds chicken cutlets, cut
   into 1-inch strips

1. Combine the coconut milk (reserving 1 tablespoon if making Peanut Dipping Sauce), cilantro, lime juice, jalapeño, garlic, salt, and pepper in a bowl and mix well. Add the chicken, stirring to coat. Cover and refrigerate for at least 20 minutes and up to 1 hour. Preheat the broiler.

2. Thread the chicken onto metal skewers, shaking off excess marinade, and broil, turning once, for 7 minutes, or until the chicken is lightly browned and cooked through. Transfer to a platter and serve immediately.

PER SERVING
carbs: 4 grams; Net Carbs: 3 grams;
fiber: 1 gram; protein: 41 grams; fat: 23 grams; calories: 387

PHASES 1−4

CHICKEN WITH CUCUMBERS

This lightly spiced chicken has a subtle flavor that makes it especially pleasing as a warm-weather meal.

PREP TIME: 10 MINUTES • COOK TIME: 20 MINUTES
4 SERVINGS

2 tablespoons butter

2 tablespoons olive oil

8 boneless chicken thighs, halved

2 small cucumbers, peeled, seeded, and chopped

2 cloves garlic, minced

salt and pepper to taste

1 cup reduced-sodium chicken broth

⅓ cup sour cream

1 tablespoon chopped fresh dill

1. Heat the butter and oil in a skillet over medium heat until hot but not smoking. Add the chicken and cook, turning frequently, for 10–12 minutes, until golden. Transfer the chicken to a plate and keep warm.

2. Add the cucumbers, garlic, salt, and pepper to the skillet, and cook, stirring frequently, for 2 minutes.

3. Return the chicken to the skillet and add the chicken broth. Bring to a boil, then simmer for 5 minutes. Remove from the heat and stir in the sour cream and dill. Serve immediately.

PER SERVING
carbs: 4.5 grams; Net Carbs: 3.5 grams;
fiber: 1 gram; protein: 33 grams; fat: 44 grams; calories: 551

PHASES 1–4

CHICKEN PAPRIKA

The first time I made this dish, Dr. Atkins was enchanted and full of praise. I hope you receive the same kudos when you serve it.

PREP TIME: 10 MINUTES • COOK TIME: 20 MINUTES

4 SERVINGS

2 tablespoons butter

¼ cup olive oil, divided

1 cup finely chopped onion

1 chicken (about 3 pounds), cut into 8 to 12 pieces

1 tablespoon Hungarian paprika (available at specialty-food stores)

salt and pepper to taste

¼ cup reduced-sodium chicken broth

¼ cup white wine

½ cup sour cream

1 large egg yolk

1. Heat the butter and 2 tablespoons of olive oil in a skillet over medium-high heat. Add the onion and cook for 3 minutes. Add the chicken pieces, skin side down, and cook for 5 minutes on each side. Add the paprika, salt, pepper, and remaining 2 tablespoons of olive oil, and cook, stirring, for 2 minutes.

2. Bring the chicken broth and wine to a boil in a small saucepan. Whisk together the sour cream and egg yolk in a bowl. Slowly add the broth-wine mixture to the egg mixture, whisking until smooth.

3. Pour the sauce over the chicken in the skillet. Cover and simmer for 10 minutes. Serve immediately.

PER SERVING

carbs: 6 grams; Net Carbs: 5 grams;
fiber: 1 gram; protein: 60 grams; fat: 59 grams; calories: 812

PHASES 1—4

CHICKEN WITH INDIAN SPICES

*W*hen simmered in turmeric, also known as Indian saffron, chicken breasts become wonderfully aromatic. Turmeric has been revered for centuries, not only for its flavor but also for its medicinal properties.

PREP TIME: 10 MINUTES • COOK TIME: 15 MINUTES
4 SERVINGS

3 tablespoons butter

1½ pounds chicken cutlets, cut
   into 1-inch strips

8 cloves garlic, minced

3 teaspoons cumin

2 teaspoons turmeric

1 teaspoon dried red pepper flakes
   (optional)

1 cup reduced-sodium chicken
   broth

1 cup whole-milk yogurt

2 tablespoons chopped cilantro or
   fresh flat-leaf parsley for garnish
   (optional)

1. Heat the butter in a large, heavy casserole over medium-high heat until the foam subsides. Add the chicken strips and cook, stirring, until browned, about 2 minutes. Add the garlic, cumin, turmeric, and the optional red pepper flakes, and cook, stirring occasionally, for 2 minutes.

2. Add the chicken broth, reduce the heat, and simmer, stirring occasionally, for about 5 minutes, until the chicken is just cooked through. Gradually stir in the yogurt and simmer very gently for 3 minutes, or until heated through (do not let it boil).

3. Transfer the chicken and sauce to a serving plate, garnish with cilantro or parsley if desired, and serve immediately.

PER SERVING
carbs: 6.5 grams; Net Carbs: 5.5 grams;
fiber: 1 gram; protein: 42 grams; fat: 13 grams; calories: 323

PHASES 3 AND 4

CREAMED CHICKEN WITH MUSHROOMS

A comforting food for cold nights, this creamed chicken is delicious on its own, or serve it on toast points made from low carb bread.

PREP TIME: 10 MINUTES • COOK TIME: 25 MINUTES
4 SERVINGS

1½ pounds chicken cutlets, cut
  into 1-inch pieces
salt and pepper to taste
2 teaspoons chopped fresh thyme or
  ½ teaspoon crumbled dried
  thyme
3 tablespoons butter, divided
2 cups sliced mushrooms

¼ cup minced shallots
⅔ cup dry white wine
⅔ cup reduced-sodium chicken
  broth
⅔ cup heavy cream
¼ cup chopped fresh flat-leaf
  parsley

1. Season the chicken with salt, pepper, and thyme. Heat 2 tablespoons of the butter in a skillet until the foam subsides. Add the chicken and cook over medium-high heat for about 3 minutes, until light golden.

2. Add the mushrooms and cook for 2 minutes, stirring occasionally. Transfer the chicken-mushroom mixture to a plate and keep warm.

3. Melt the remaining 1 tablespoon of butter in the skillet over medium heat. Add the shallots and cook for 2 minutes. Stir in the wine and broth, scraping up any browned bits from the bottom of the pan, and bring to a boil. Reduce the heat and simmer for 5 minutes. Add the cream and gently simmer for 5 minutes.

4. Return the chicken-mushroom mixture to the skillet, stir in the parsley, and heat through. Serve immediately.

PER SERVING
carbs: 5 grams; Net Carbs: 4.5 grams;
fiber: 0.5 gram; protein: 42 grams; fat: 26 grams; calories: 447

PHASES 1–4

TOMATILLO CHICKEN

*W*hen I want a quick weeknight meal, I often prepare chicken. With a jar of green salsa in the cupboard, this delicious entrée comes together in no time.

PREP TIME: 10 MINUTES • COOK TIME: 45 MINUTES
4 SERVINGS

CHICKEN

1 tablespoon olive oil

¾ teaspoon salt

1 teaspoon cumin

4 large whole chicken legs

1 cup roasted tomatillo salsa, mild
   or medium

½ cup reduced-sodium chicken
   broth

GARNISH

½ teaspoon olive oil

¼ cup pumpkin seeds

¼ teaspoon salt

1. Place a rack in the top third of the oven (about 6 inches from the heat source). Preheat the oven to 350°F.

2. Heat the oil in a 12-inch ovenproof skillet over medium-high heat. Combine the salt and cumin and sprinkle evenly on both sides of the chicken. Brown the legs 6 minutes per side, turning once, until deep golden (do not let the chicken burn; reduce heat slightly if it gets too dark).

3. Add salsa and broth, and cover loosely with foil. Bake for 35 minutes.

4. Meanwhile, prepare the garnish. Heat the oil in a small skillet. Add the pumpkin seeds and cook, shaking the pan, for 1 to 2 minutes, until the seeds are lightly toasted and slightly puffed (seeds may pop). Sprinkle with the salt and set aside.

5. Uncover chicken and bake 5–6 minutes more, until deeply browned.

6. Transfer the chicken to a platter, spoon the juices over the chicken, and sprinkle with the pumpkin seeds. Serve immediately.

PER SERVING
carbs: 9.5 grams; Net Carbs: 6.5 grams;
fiber: 3 grams; protein: 48 grams; fat: 2.5 grams; calories: 525

PHASES 2–4

BREAST OF DUCK WITH RED WINE SAUCE

*S*liced duck drizzled with this rich creamy wine sauce creates a sophisticated main course for a formal dinner.

PREP TIME: 10 MINUTES • COOK TIME: 25 MINUTES
4 SERVINGS

2 whole boneless duck breasts

2 tablespoons butter

2 large shallots, finely chopped

1 cup dry red wine

2 tablespoons balsamic vinegar

2 tablespoons Worcestershire sauce

2 beef bouillon cubes

½ cup heavy cream

1. Prick the duck skin all over with a fork. Heat a nonstick skillet over medium-high heat until hot. Place the duck breasts, skin side down, in the skillet and cook for 8–10 minutes, or until the skin is crisp and brown. Turn the duck and cook for another 5 minutes. Transfer the duck to a plate and keep warm.

2. Wipe out the skillet. Melt the butter over medium heat. Add the shallots and cook about 1 minute, until barely golden. Add the wine, vinegar, Worcestershire sauce, and bouillon cubes, and bring to a boil, stirring to dissolve the cubes. Reduce the heat and simmer for 5 minutes. Stir in the cream and heat through (do not let it boil).

3. Cut the duck into thin slices and then pour the sauce on top. Serve immediately.

PER SERVING
carbs: 6.5 grams; Net Carbs: 6.5 grams;
fiber: 0 grams; protein: 19 grams; fat: 20.5 grams; calories: 323

PHASES 1–4

PORK

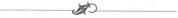

Pork Chops with Orange and Rosemary

Pork with Chili Sauce

Stir-Fried Pork with Water Chestnuts

Garlic-Dill Meatballs

Ham with Port Cream Sauce

Barbecued Spareribs

Pork Casserole with Tomatoes and Mushrooms

Pork Chops with Poblano Pepper and Onion
Cream Sauce

Boneless Pork Chops with Spicy Rub

PORK CHOPS WITH ORANGE AND ROSEMARY

*I*n this recipe, orange and mustard enliven the flavor of pork chops. The sauce is so sweet and tangy that you'll never miss the more traditional apple-sauce accompaniment.

PREP TIME: 5 MINUTES • COOK TIME: 12 MINUTES
4 SERVINGS

4 center-cut pork chops, about
 ¾ inch thick
salt and pepper to taste
¼ cup Atkins Quick Quisine™
 Bake Mix or soy flour
2 tablespoons plus 1 teaspoon
 butter, divided

¼ cup chopped shallots
⅔ cup dry white wine
1 teaspoon Worcestershire sauce
1 tablespoon grated orange zest
2 teaspoons Dijon mustard
1 teaspoon crumbled dried
 rosemary

1. Season the pork chops with salt and pepper and lightly dust with the bake mix, shaking off any excess.

2. Heat 2 tablespoons of butter in a skillet over medium-high heat and cook the pork chops for 5 minutes on each side. Transfer the pork chops to a serving platter and keep warm.

3. Heat the remaining 1 teaspoon of butter and cook the shallots until they become softened, about 1 minute. Add the wine, Worcestershire sauce, orange zest, mustard, and rosemary. Bring to a boil, then lower the heat and simmer for 2 minutes, scraping up any brown bits on the bottom of the skillet. Pour the sauce over the pork chops and serve immediately.

PER SERVING
carbs: 5.5 grams; Net Carbs: 4.5 grams;
fiber: 1 gram; protein: 47 grams; fat: 29 grams; calories: 503

PHASES 1–4

PORK WITH CHILI SAUCE

*S*errano chili gives this dish a wonderful Southwestern flavor. You can use beef instead of pork for an equally tasty variation.

PREP TIME: 5 MINUTES • COOK TIME: 20 MINUTES
4 SERVINGS

1 scallion, chopped

3 cloves garlic

½ cup chopped green pepper

½ cup chopped tomatillos or
  green tomatoes

1 serrano chili, seeded and
  chopped

½ cup beef stock

1 tablespoon fresh lime juice

3 tablespoons olive oil

1½ pounds pork loin, cubed

1 tablespoon chili powder

1. Preheat the broiler. Combine the scallion, garlic, pepper, tomatillos, chili, stock, and lime juice in a food processor and process for 1 minute, or until well blended.

2. Transfer the mixture to a saucepan and bring to a boil. Reduce the heat and simmer for 10 minutes.

3. Heat the oil in a large nonstick skillet over medium heat. Add the pork and sprinkle with the chili powder. Cook for 6–8 minutes, until browned and cooked through. Pour off the excess oil. Add the chili sauce to the skillet and mix well. Transfer to a platter and serve immediately.

PER SERVING
carbs: 5 grams; Net Carbs: 3.5 grams;
fiber: 1.5 grams; protein: 38 grams; fat: 19 grams; calories: 347

PHASES 1–4

STIR-FRIED PORK WITH WATER CHESTNUTS

*C*runchy water chestnuts add lots of texture to this simple stir-fry with an Asian flair.

PREP TIME: 15 MINUTES • COOK TIME: 15 MINUTES
4 SERVINGS

2 tablespoons canola oil

1½ pounds pork loin, sliced into
  thin strips

4 scallions, cut in ½-inch pieces

3 cloves garlic, minced

1 cup sliced water chestnuts,
  drained and patted dry

⅔ cup sliced mushrooms

½ green pepper, cut into thin strips

2 tablespoons rice wine vinegar

salt and pepper to taste

1 tablespoon sesame oil

1 tablespoon soy sauce

1. Heat the canola oil in a heavy skillet or wok. Add the pork and stir-fry for 3–4 minutes, until the pork begins to brown. Add the scallions and garlic and cook for 1 minute more. Add the water chestnuts, mushrooms, and pepper. Cook, stirring, for 2 minutes.

2. Add the vinegar, salt, pepper, sesame oil, and soy sauce, and cook for 2 minutes. Serve immediately.

PER SERVING
carbs: 7 grams; Net Carbs: 5.5 grams;
fiber: 1.5 grams; protein: 34 grams; fat: 23 grams; calories: 368

PHASES 1–4

GARLIC-DILL MEATBALLS

Ever since I prepared this for a dinner party, I get requests for encores. Serve the meatballs with toothpicks for an hors d'oeuvre or on a bed of Creamy Mushroom Sauce (page 158) as an entrée or first course.

PREP TIME: 20 MINUTES • COOK TIME: 35 MINUTES
2 ENTRÉE SERVINGS OR 4 APPETIZER SERVINGS

1 pound ground chicken
½ pound ground pork
1 small onion, finely chopped
½ cup ground pork rinds (optional)
1 egg

2 cloves garlic, minced
2 tablespoons chopped fresh dill
salt and pepper to taste
2 tablespoons canola oil

1. Preheat the oven to 375°F. Combine the chicken, pork, onion, pork rinds if using, egg, garlic, dill, salt, and pepper in a bowl and mix well. Divide the mixture into twelve 2-inch meatballs.

2. Heat the oil in a large ovenproof skillet over medium-high heat until hot but not smoking. Brown the meatballs on all sides, about 6 minutes.

3. Transfer the skillet to the oven and bake, covered, for 15 minutes, until cooked through. Serve immediately.

PER SERVING
carbs: 4.5 grams; Net Carbs: 3.5 grams;
fiber: 1 gram; protein: 70.5 grams; fat: 39.5 grams; calories: 671

PHASES 1–4

HAM WITH PORT CREAM SAUCE

You won't believe how easy it is to dress up convenient precooked ham steaks with this rich port sauce. You can also use leftover ham in this dish and achieve great results.

PREP TIME: 15 MINUTES • COOK TIME: 15 MINUTES
4 SERVINGS

2 tablespoons butter
¼ cup finely chopped shallots
⅓ cup dry white wine
¼ cup port wine
2 pounds reduced-sodium cooked
   ham steaks

⅓ cup heavy cream
1 teaspoon tomato paste
salt and pepper to taste

1. Heat the butter in a skillet over medium heat until the foam subsides. Add the shallots and cook until translucent, about 2 minutes. Add the white wine, port, and ham to the skillet. Bring to a boil, then lower the heat and simmer for 3 minutes. Transfer the ham to a serving plate and keep warm.

2. Whisk the cream and tomato paste into the skillet sauce and bring to a gentle boil. Lower the heat slightly and simmer for about 4 minutes, until slightly thickened. Season with salt and pepper. Pour the sauce over the ham and serve immediately.

PER SERVING
carbs: 5 grams; Net Carbs: 5 grams;
fiber: 0 grams; protein: 38.5 grams; fat: 20.5 grams; calories: 386

PHASES 1–4

BARBECUED SPARERIBS

*R*ibs *are one of my favorite indulgences, so I created a quick version that you can put together in a pinch, even after a long day at work.*

PREP TIME: 10 MINUTES • COOK TIME: 25 MINUTES
4 SERVINGS

3 pounds spareribs

2 bay leaves

2 tablespoons whole peppercorns

2 tablespoons butter, softened

2 tablespoons Atkins Quick Quisine™ Barbeque Sauce

2 teaspoons hot pepper sauce

1. Preheat the broiler.

2. Place the ribs in a large pot, cover with water, add the bay leaves and peppercorns, and bring to a boil. Lower the heat, cover, and simmer for 20 minutes.

3. Meanwhile, combine the butter, barbecue sauce, and hot pepper sauce in a small bowl. Drain the ribs. Pat the butter mixture all over the ribs.

4. Broil the ribs for 4–6 minutes, turning once, or until browned and crisp. Serve immediately.

PER SERVING
carbs: 3 grams; Net Carbs: 1.5 grams;
fiber: 1.5 grams; protein: 47 grams; fat: 54.5 grams; calories: 700

PHASES 1–4

PORK CASSEROLE WITH TOMATOES AND MUSHROOMS

*Y*ou don't have to wait for hours to savor this hearty casserole, enriched with a flavorful, tomato-mushroom sauce. It's ready in less than 40 minutes.

PREP TIME: 10 MINUTES • COOK TIME: 25 MINUTES
4 SERVINGS

2 tablespoons olive oil

4 center-cut boneless pork chops, each sliced against the grain into 3 pieces

2 onions, chopped

2 tomatoes, chopped

¾ cup sliced white mushrooms

3 cloves garlic, minced

½ cup reduced-sodium chicken broth

salt and pepper to taste

⅓ cup pitted black olives (optional)

1. Heat the oil in a large, heavy skillet over medium-high heat until hot but not smoking. Add the pork pieces and cook for 2 minutes on each side. Transfer to a plate and keep warm.

2. Add the onions to the skillet and cook, stirring, for 3 minutes. Stir in the tomatoes, mushrooms, and garlic, and cook for 3 minutes. Add the chicken broth, salt, and pepper, and bring to a boil. Reduce the heat, cover, and simmer, stirring occasionally, for 10 minutes.

3. Return the pork to the pan and cook, uncovered, for 2 minutes to heat through. Stir in the olives, if using, and simmer for 3 minutes. Serve immediately.

PER SERVING
carbs: 9 grams; Net Carbs: 7 grams;
fiber: 2 grams; protein: 20 grams; fat: 12 grams; calories: 225

PHASES 1–4

PORK CHOPS WITH POBLANO PEPPER AND ONION CREAM SAUCE

In Mexico, poblano chili peppers are roasted, then peeled. Here, I've omitted those steps, but the final result remains scrumptious.

PREP TIME: 10 MINUTES • COOK TIME: 15 MINUTES
4 SERVINGS

1 tablespoon olive oil

4 center-cut pork chops (about
   10 ounces each)

salt and pepper to taste

1 cup seeded and chopped poblano
   chilies

1 cup chopped yellow onion

1 cup heavy cream

¼ cup water

1. Heat the olive oil in a large skillet over medium-high heat until hot but not smoking. Season the pork chops with salt and pepper, and cook for 4–5 minutes on each side, until golden brown. Transfer the chops to a plate and keep warm.

2. Reduce the heat to medium-low. Add the poblano chilies, onion, salt, and pepper, and cook, stirring occasionally, for 6–7 minutes. Stir in the cream and water and bring to a simmer. Add the pork chops and cook for 2 minutes on each side.

3. Transfer the pork to a serving platter and pour the cream sauce on top. Serve immediately.

PER SERVING
carbs: 7.5 grams; Net Carbs: 6 grams;
fiber: 1.5 grams; protein: 45.5 grams; fat: 37.5 grams; calories: 557

PHASES 1–4

BONELESS PORK CHOPS WITH
SPICY RUB

A quick and flavorful spice rub adds punch to pork. Serve this dish with
green salsa and low carb tortillas.

PREP TIME: 10 MINUTES • CHILL TIME: 15 MINUTES
COOK TIME: 12 MINUTES
4 SERVINGS

2 tablespoons olive oil

1 tablespoon chili powder

1 teaspoon hot paprika

1 teaspoon minced garlic

1 teaspoon salt

½ teaspoon crumbled dried
oregano

¼ teaspoon ground cumin

¼ teaspoon freshly ground black
pepper

4 boneless pork chops
(8 to 10 ounces each)

1 lime, cut into 8 wedges

1. In a small bowl, combine the olive oil, chili powder, paprika, garlic,
salt, oregano, cumin, and pepper. Mix well. Rub the spice mixture evenly
over the pork chops. Cover and refrigerate for 15 minutes.

2. Heat the broiler. Broil the pork chops for 5 to 6 minutes on each
side, until nicely browned and cooked through. Serve immediately, with
2 wedges of lime for each chop.

PER SERVING
carbs: 2 grams; Net Carbs: 1 gram;
fiber: 1 gram; protein: 48.5 grams; fat: 25 grams; calories: 438

PHASES 1–4

LAMB

Broiled Marinated Lamb Chops
Grilled Lemon and Rosemary Lamb Kebobs
Rack of Lamb with Brussels Sprouts
Lamb Curry
Lamb Paprikash with Cabbage

BROILED MARINATED LAMB CHOPS

*S*imple and scrumptious, these lamb chops burst with the zesty flavor of the marinade, which also gives them a wonderful glazelike crust.

PREP TIME: 10 MINUTES • MARINATE TIME: 15 MINUTES
COOK TIME: 8 MINUTES
4 SERVINGS

2 tablespoons olive oil

1 tablespoon Worcestershire sauce

3 tablespoons fresh lime juice

3 tablespoons soy sauce

3 cloves garlic, minced

salt and pepper to taste

2 pounds lamb chops (each about
¾ inch thick)

1. Preheat the broiler. Whisk together the oil, Worcestershire sauce, lime juice, soy sauce, garlic, salt, and pepper in a large bowl. Add the lamb chops and let them marinate, covered, in the refrigerator for 15 minutes and up to 1 hour.

2. Remove the lamb chops from the marinade and pat dry. Broil the chops for 4 minutes on each side for medium-rare, or until desired doneness. Serve immediately.

PER SERVING
carbs: 1 gram; Net Carbs: 1 gram;
fiber: 0 grams; protein: 30.5 grams; fat: 11.5 grams; calories: 237

PHASES 1—4

GRILLED LEMON AND
ROSEMARY LAMB KEBOBS

*L*amb was one of Dr. Atkins' favorite dishes, and this rendition could not be simpler. The marinade coats each piece of lamb, making it succulent and flavorful. If you do not have a grill, you can cook the lamb under the broiler.

PREP TIME: 10 MINUTES • MARINATE TIME: 15 MINUTES
COOK TIME: 12 MINUTES
4 SERVINGS

¼ cup fresh lemon juice

¼ cup olive oil

1 tablespoon chopped fresh
    rosemary or 1 teaspoon dried
    rosemary

2 cloves garlic, minced

1 teaspoon grated lemon zest

2 pounds boneless lamb chops,
    cut into 1-inch cubes

1. Preheat the grill or broiler. Whisk together the lemon juice, oil, rosemary, garlic, and lemon zest in a bowl. Add the lamb and toss gently, making sure each piece is well coated. Cover and refrigerate for 10–15 minutes.

2. Thread the lamb onto skewers. Grill or broil, turning once, for 12 minutes for medium doneness. Serve immediately.

PER SERVING
carbs: 0.5 gram; Net Carbs: 0.5 gram;
fiber: 0 grams; protein: 47 grams; fat: 18.5 grams; calories: 372

PHASES 1–4

RACK OF LAMB WITH BRUSSELS SPROUTS

*D*ramatic rack of lamb is a perfect entrée for a special occasion. You can double or triple the recipe for an elegant dinner party.

PREP TIME: 30 MINUTES • COOK TIME: 35 MINUTES
4 SERVINGS

1 pint stemmed fresh brussels
   sprouts, quartered
2 tablespoons olive oil
two 1-pound racks of lamb (about
   6 ribs each), cut in half
1 tablespoon Dijon mustard
1 tablespoon coriander seeds

1 tablespoon chopped fresh
   rosemary or 1½ teaspoons
   crumbled dried rosemary
1 tablespoon black peppercorns
2 cloves garlic
salt to taste

1. Preheat the oven to 425°F. Place the brussels sprouts in a roasting pan and sprinkle with the oil. Brush the lamb with the mustard.

2. Place the coriander, rosemary, peppercorns, and garlic in a food processor and process for 10 seconds. Pat the lamb with the herb mixture, coating thoroughly, then sprinkle with the salt.

3. Arrange the lamb on top of the brussels sprouts and roast 25 minutes for rare, 30–35 minutes for medium doneness. Serve immediately.

PER SERVING
carbs: 7 grams; Net Carbs: 5 grams;
fiber: 2 grams; protein: 28 grams; fat: 43 grams; calories: 523

PHASES 1–4

LAMB CURRY

When lamb is braised with spices, it becomes infused with flavor. This dish is made with the neck of the lamb, an inexpensive but extremely tender cut. The tasty lamb requires only 30 minutes of braising, but if you have the time, you can braise it for up to an hour for added flavor.

PREP TIME: 25 MINUTES • COOK TIME: 30 MINUTES
4 SERVINGS

1 tablespoon olive oil

2 pounds neck of lamb, cut into 2-inch pieces, or 1½ pounds lamb shoulder, cut into 1-inch cubes

2 tablespoons Atkins Quick Quisine™ Bake Mix or soy flour

2 teaspoons curry powder

1 teaspoon ground cumin

1 teaspoon ground coriander

3 cloves garlic, minced

½ cup reduced-sodium chicken broth

2 tablespoons fresh lemon juice

½ cup whole-milk yogurt

salt to taste

1. Heat the oil in a large casserole over medium-high heat until hot but not smoking. Dust the lamb with the bake mix. Add the lamb to the pot and cook in a single layer for 3–4 minutes on each side, or until browned. Stir in the curry, cumin, coriander, and garlic; then stir in the chicken broth and lemon juice. Cover the casserole tightly and braise over low heat for 30 minutes.

2. Stir in the yogurt and salt during the last 5 minutes of cooking. Do not boil. Serve immediately.

PER SERVING
carbs: 5 grams; Net Carbs: 4 grams;
fiber: 1 gram; protein: 28 grams; fat: 24 grams; calories: 348

PHASES 2–4

LAMB PAPRIKASH WITH CABBAGE

*C*abbage *becomes very sweet when it is simmered. In this dish the cabbage lends a wonderful flavor to the lamb.*

PREP TIME: 20 MINUTES • COOK TIME: 20 MINUTES
4 SERVINGS

2 tablespoons olive oil

1 tablespoon butter

2 pounds lamb shoulder, cut into
   2-inch cubes

1 tablespoon paprika

½ head cabbage, thinly sliced
   (about 3 cups)

½ cup chopped onion

3 cloves garlic, minced

1 teaspoon caraway seeds

¼ cup reduced-sodium chicken
   broth

¼ cup heavy cream

salt and pepper to taste

1. Heat the oil and butter in a large, heavy skillet over medium heat until the foam subsides. Add the lamb and paprika, and brown the lamb on all sides, for about 8 minutes. Transfer the lamb to a plate.

2. Add the cabbage, onion, garlic, and caraway seeds to the skillet, and cook for 2 minutes, stirring occasionally. Place the lamb on top of cabbage mixture, add the broth, and bring to a boil. Lower the heat, cover, and simmer for 5 minutes.

3. Stir in the cream, salt, and pepper, and cook, uncovered, for 2 minutes. Serve immediately.

PER SERVING
carbs: 7.5 grams; Net Carbs: 5 grams;
fiber: 2.5 grams; protein: 33.5 grams; fat: 40.5 grams; calories: 532

PHASES 1−4

VEAL

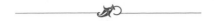

Veal Scallops with Wine and Mushrooms

Veal Saltimbocca

Veal Burgers

Veal Chops Smothered in Browned
Butter-Sage Mushrooms

VEAL SCALLOPS WITH
WINE AND MUSHROOMS

The tang of lemon and the earthiness of sautéed mushrooms complement these delicate veal scallops. Try serving them with Sautéed Zucchini with Nutmeg (page 134).

(page 134)

PREP TIME: 15 MINUTES • COOK TIME: 15 MINUTES
4 SERVINGS

2 tablespoons butter

2 tablespoons olive oil

2 cups thinly sliced mushrooms

⅓ cup chopped scallions

1¼ pounds veal scallops, pounded
⅛ inch thick

½ cup dry white wine

4 teaspoons fresh lemon juice

salt and pepper to taste

1. Heat 1 tablespoon of the butter and 1 tablespoon of the oil in a large skillet over medium-high heat until the foam subsides. Add the mushrooms and scallions, and cook, stirring occasionally, until softened, about 5 minutes. Transfer with a slotted spoon to a bowl.

2. Add half of the veal to the skillet and cook for 1 minute on each side. Transfer the veal to a plate and keep warm. Heat the remaining 1 tablespoon each of butter and oil in the skillet, add the remaining veal, and cook in the same manner. Transfer the veal to a plate.

3. Add the wine, lemon juice, reserved mushrooms and scallions, salt, and pepper to the skillet. Bring to a boil, then lower the heat and simmer for 2 minutes. Pour the sauce over the veal and serve immediately.

PER SERVING
carbs: 2.5 grams; Net Carbs: 2 grams;
fiber: 0.5 gram; protein: 34 grams; fat: 16.5 grams; calories: 317

PHASES 1–4

VEAL SALTIMBOCCA

Here's a delicious Italian classic that's easy to prepare and makes a lovely presentation.

PREP TIME: 25 MINUTES • COOK TIME: 15 MINUTES
4 SERVINGS

1 pound veal scallops, pounded
⅛ inch thick
salt and pepper to taste
½ cup Atkins Quick Quisine™
  Bake Mix or soy flour
4 tablespoons butter, divided
¼ cup freshly grated Parmesan
  cheese

4 thin slices prosciutto
⅓ cup dry white wine
1 tablespoon Worcestershire sauce
½ tablespoon chopped fresh sage or
  ¾ teaspoon crumbled dried sage

1. Preheat the oven to 375°F. Season the veal with salt and pepper and dredge in the bake mix, shaking off any excess.

2. Heat 2 tablespoons of the butter in a large skillet over medium-high heat until the foam subsides. Add half of the veal and cook for 1 minute on each side. Transfer the veal to a baking sheet. Repeat with 1 more tablespoon of butter and the remaining veal.

3. Sprinkle the Parmesan evenly over the veal and top each scallop with a piece of prosciutto, cut to fit the size of the veal. Bake for 5 minutes.

4. Add the wine, Worcestershire sauce, and sage to the skillet. Bring to a boil, scraping up any browned bits from the bottom of the skillet. Lower the heat and simmer for 2 minutes. Remove from the heat and whisk in the remaining 1 tablespoon of butter.

5. Transfer the veal to a serving plate, pour the sauce over it, and serve immediately.

PER SERVING
carbs: 4 grams; Net Carbs: 2.5 grams;
fiber: 1.5 grams; protein: 39 grams; fat: 18 grams; calories: 352

PHASES 1–4

VEAL BURGERS

*I*nstead of beef burgers, try these veal burgers for a change of pace. Cilantro and green salsa add zip.

PREP TIME: 10 MINUTES • COOK TIME: 10 MINUTES

4 SERVINGS

1½ pounds ground veal

2 scallions, finely chopped

2 tablespoons chopped fresh
  cilantro

2 tablespoons green salsa

½ teaspoon chili powder

salt and pepper to taste

1 tablespoon canola oil

1. In a large bowl, mix the veal, scallions, cilantro, salsa, chili powder, salt, and pepper. Gently shape the mixture into 4 patties.

2. Heat the oil in a large nonstick skillet over medium heat until very hot. Cook the patties 4–5 minutes on each side, until cooked through. Serve with extra green salsa.

PER SERVING

carbs: 0.5 gram; Net Carbs: 0.5 gram;

fiber: 0 grams; protein: 24.5 grams; fat: 11 grams; calories: 208

PHASES 1–4

VEAL CHOPS SMOTHERED IN BROWNED BUTTER-SAGE MUSHROOMS

I love this recipe! The combination of flavors is wonderful. Fresh sage is crisped in butter and used as a garnish, and its flavorful butter is used to sauté the mushrooms.

PREP TIME: 10 MINUTES • COOK TIME: 25 MINUTES
4 SERVINGS

---

4 tablespoons butter
12 fresh sage leaves
1 pound sliced mushrooms, such as
   white button, oyster, shiitake
salt and pepper to taste

4 loin or rib veal chops (about
   12 ounces each), 1¼ to
   1½ inches thick
2 tablespoons olive oil

1. In a large skillet over medium-high heat, melt the butter. When the butter stops bubbling, add the sage leaves. Cook for 1 minute, until lightly crisp. Remove the sage with a slotted spoon and transfer to paper towels to drain.

2. Add the mushrooms to the skillet and sprinkle with salt and pepper. Cook, stirring frequently, about 5 minutes, until lightly browned and most of the liquid has evaporated. Transfer to a plate and cover with foil to keep warm.

3. Rinse out the skillet. Season the veal chops with salt and pepper. Heat the olive oil over medium-high heat. Add the veal chops and cook for 10–15 minutes, until the internal temperature registers between 120° and 125°F on an instant-read thermometer. Remove the chops from the skillet and cover with foil.

4. Return the mushrooms to the skillet. Cook for 3 minutes to warm through. Serve the chops smothered with mushrooms. Garnish with the sage leaves.

PER SERVING
carbs: 4.5 grams; Net Carbs: 4 grams;
fiber: 0.5 gram; protein: 86.5 grams; fat: 32.5 grams; calories: 673

PHASES 1−4

BEEF

Quick & Easy Beef Goulash
Chevapchichi (Spicy Meat Rolls)
Beef Burgers with Feta and Tomato
Steak au Poivre
Rib-Eye Steak with Red Wine Sauce
Spiced Skirt Steak

Quick & Easy Beef Goulash

*W*hen I succeeded in developing a recipe for a quick beef goulash, I was thrilled. And even though this stew takes only an hour, it still has that rich braised flavor.

PREP TIME: 30 MINUTES • COOK TIME: 30 MINUTES
4 SERVINGS

2 large tomatoes

4 scallions

5 large cloves garlic

⅓ cup olive oil

3 pounds boneless beef sirloin,
  cut into ¾-inch cubes

1 tablespoon paprika

salt and pepper to taste

½ cup heavy cream

1 cup reduced-sodium beef broth

1. Combine the tomatoes, scallions, and garlic in a food processor and purée until smooth, about 1 minute. Heat 2 tablespoons of the oil in a saucepan over medium heat until hot but not smoking. Add the tomato mixture and cook, stirring occasionally, for 8 minutes.

2. Season the beef with the paprika, salt, and pepper. Heat the remaining 3½ tablespoons of oil in a large, deep skillet over medium-high heat until hot but not smoking. Add the meat in batches and cook until browned, 5–7 minutes per batch.

3. Pour the tomato mixture over the meat and cook over medium-high heat, stirring occasionally, for 30 minutes. Stir in the cream and beef broth, and cook for 2 minutes, or until heated through (do not let the goulash boil). Serve immediately.

PER SERVING
carbs: 9 grams; Net Carbs: 7 grams;
fiber: 2 grams; protein: 82 grams; fat: 50 grams; calories: 828

PHASES 1–4

CHEVAPCHICHI (SPICY MEAT ROLLS)

They're not your mother's meatballs. Flavorful and rich, these hot and spicy meat rolls pair nicely with refreshing chilled Cucumber-Dill Sauce (page 151).

PREP TIME: 20 MINUTES • COOK TIME: 15 MINUTES
4 SERVINGS

½ pound ground veal
½ pound ground beef
½ pound ground pork
½ medium onion, finely chopped
2 cloves garlic, minced
2 tablespoons club soda

1 tablespoon finely chopped fresh
    flat-leaf parsley
1 teaspoon Hungarian paprika
½ teaspoon freshly ground pepper
2 tablespoons olive oil
salt to taste

1. Combine the veal, beef, pork, onion, garlic, club soda, parsley, paprika, and pepper in a large bowl and mix well. Take 1 heaping tablespoon of the mixture and shape it into a 3-inch ball. Continue making balls in the same manner until all the mixture is used (you will have 15 to 20 balls).

2. Heat the oil in a heavy skillet over medium heat until hot but not smoking. Reduce heat to medium. Cook the meatballs in batches, turning frequently, for 12–15 minutes, until nicely browned and cooked through. Season the meatballs with salt and serve immediately.

PER SERVING
carbs: 2 grams; Net Carbs: 1.5 grams;
fiber: 0.5 gram; protein: 29 grams; fat: 26.5 grams; calories: 370

PHASES 1–4

Beef Burgers with Feta and Tomato

$\mathcal{T}$hink of these burgers as mini meatloaves with lots of flavor. They are great on the grill and equally delicious panfried.

PREP TIME: 15 MINUTES • COOK TIME: 10 MINUTES
4 SERVINGS

2 pounds ground beef (round or
    chuck)
1 cup chopped fresh spinach
1 cup chopped tomato
4 ounces crumbled feta cheese
2 scallions (white part only),
    chopped

3 teaspoons chopped fresh thyme or
    1 teaspoon crumbled dried
    thyme
salt and pepper to taste
2 teaspoons chopped fresh mint
    (optional)

1. Combine all the ingredients in a large bowl and mix well. Form the meat into 4 patties.

2. Grill or panfry the patties over medium-high heat for 5 minutes on each side for medium-rare, or until desired doneness. Serve immediately.

PER SERVING
carbs: 4 grams; Net Carbs: 3 grams;
fiber: 1 gram; protein: 45.5 grams; fat: 41.5 grams; calories: 580

PHASES 1–4

STEAK AU POIVRE

*S*teak au poivre is one of the great indulgences of doing Atkins. The combination of peppercorns, cognac, and cream is sophisticated and flavorful. We have added a touch of unsweetened ketchup, which imparts a lovely color and a hint of fruitiness to this classic dish.

PREP TIME: 10 MINUTES • COOK TIME: 20 MINUTES
4 SERVINGS

¼ cup crushed mixed peppercorns
  (see Hint)
4 boneless sirloin shell steaks,
  about 1 inch thick
¼ cup olive oil

1 cup heavy cream
2 tablespoons Atkins Kitchen™
  Ketch-A-Tomato
2 tablespoons cognac
salt to taste

1. Spread the peppercorns on a work surface and press both sides of the steaks into the peppercorns to coat well.

2. Heat 2 tablespoons of the oil in a large, heavy skillet over medium-high heat until hot but not smoking. Add 2 steaks and cook for 5 minutes on each side for medium-rare doneness. Remove the steaks from the skillet and tent with foil. Repeat with the remaining 2 tablespoons of oil and 2 steaks.

3. Add the cream, ketchup, cognac, and salt to the skillet. Bring to a boil, stirring and scraping up any browned bits from the bottom of the skillet. Lower the heat and cook, stirring, for 2 minutes. Pour the sauce over the steaks and serve immediately.

PER SERVING
carbs: 6.5 grams; Net Carbs: 4.5 grams;
fiber: 2 grams; protein: 46.5 grams; fat: 50 grams; calories: 685

PHASES 1–4

HINT: To crush peppercorns, place them in a plastic bag and flatten them with a rolling pin or the flat side of a knife.

Rib-Eye Steak with Red Wine Sauce

his rich, comforting dish is perfect for the colder months. If you have access to fresh herbs, add some chopped tarragon or rosemary to the sauce.

PREP TIME: 15 MINUTES • COOK TIME: 25 MINUTES

4 SERVINGS

¼ cup olive oil

two 1-pound boneless rib-eye
    steaks, about ½ inch thick

2 tablespoons butter

4 large cloves garlic, minced

⅓ cup finely chopped shallots

1 cup red wine

½ cup reduced-sodium beef broth

½ teaspoon freshly ground pepper

salt to taste

1. Heat 2 tablespoons of the oil in a large, heavy skillet over medium-high heat until hot but not smoking. Lower the heat to medium, add one steak, and cook for 6 minutes on each side for medium. Remove the steak from the skillet and keep warm. Repeat with the remaining 2 tablespoons of oil and the second steak.

2. Add the butter to the skillet and heat until the foam subsides. Add the garlic and shallots, and cook, stirring, for about 5 minutes, until the shallots are transparent. Add the wine, broth, pepper, and salt, and bring to a boil, scraping up any browned bits from the bottom of the pan. Lower the heat and simmer for 3 minutes.

3. Slice the steaks into thin strips and top with the wine sauce. Serve immediately.

PER SERVING

carbs: 5 grams; Net Carbs: 5 grams;
fiber: 0 grams; protein: 48.5 grams; fat: 39 grams; calories: 612

PHASES 1–4

SPICED SKIRT STEAK

*S*imple and flavorful, this quick-to-fix skirt steak is a great staple for doing Atkins. Serve it with Roasted Peppers in Garlic Oil (page 138) or toss the sliced steak with baby greens and your favorite homemade dressing.

PREP TIME: ABOUT 20 MINUTES • COOK TIME: 10 MINUTES
4 SERVINGS

2 teaspoons paprika

2 teaspoons ground cumin

2 teaspoons ground coriander

salt and pepper to taste

two 1-pound skirt steaks

1. Preheat the grill or broiler. Combine the paprika, cumin, coriander, salt, and pepper in a small bowl. Rub the spice mixture over entire surface of the steaks. Cover the steaks with plastic wrap and refrigerate for 20 minutes.

2. Grill or broil the steaks for 2½–3 minutes on each side for medium-rare. Let stand for 5 minutes.

3. Cut the steaks diagonally into thin slices. Serve immediately, or refrigerate, well wrapped, for up to 2 days.

PER SERVING
carbs: 1.5 grams; Net Carbs: 0.5 gram;
fiber: 1 gram; protein: 48.5 grams; fat: 16.5 grams; calories: 359

PHASES 1–4

VEGETABLES

―――――― ✦ ――――――

Wax Beans with Garlic-Tarragon Vinaigrette
Sautéed Zucchini with Nutmeg
Cauliflower with Cumin Seed
Cauliflower–Macaroni and Cheese
Avocado–Red Pepper Purée with Garlic
Roasted Peppers in Garlic Oil
Vegetable Medley
Mixed Broiled Vegetables
Sautéed Spinach with Garlic and Olive Oil
Chiles Rellenos
Broccoli Rabe with Spicy Sausage
Broccoli Purée with Garlic
Green Beans with Anchovy Sauce
Snow Peas with Hazelnuts
Asparagus Viniagrette
Sautéed Kale with Ricotta Salata

WAX BEANS WITH
GARLIC-TARRAGON VINAIGRETTE

*W*ax *beans are wonderfully flavorful when they are tossed with this simple garlic-tarragon vinaigrette. Serve as a side dish with beef or lamb.*

PREP TIME: 10 MINUTES • COOK TIME: 5 MINUTES
4 SERVINGS

2 cups wax beans, trimmed

⅓ cup finely chopped onion

¼ cup olive oil

2 tablespoons white wine vinegar

1 clove garlic, minced

1 tablespoon chopped fresh tarragon or 1½ teaspoons crumbled dried tarragon

salt and pepper to taste

1. Bring 2 quarts of salted water to a boil in a large saucepan. Add the wax beans and cook for 5–6 minutes, until tender. Drain the beans and refresh under cold water to stop cooking.

2. In a small bowl, whisk together the onion, olive oil, vinegar, garlic, tarragon, salt, and pepper.

3. Put the wax beans in a serving bowl. Pour the vinaigrette over them and toss well. Let the beans stand for 10 minutes. Serve immediately, or refrigerate, in an airtight container, for up to 1 day.

PER SERVING
carbs: 11.5 grams; Net Carbs: 9.5 grams;
fiber: 2 grams; protein: 13.5 grams; fat: 13.5 grams; calories: 169

PHASES 2–4

SAUTÉED ZUCCHINI WITH NUTMEG

Freshly grated nutmeg is delightfully pungent, and it is fun to use. Try it instead of the ground kind.

PREP TIME: 5 MINUTES • COOK TIME: 10 MINUTES
4 SERVINGS

2 tablespoons butter

2 medium zucchini, cut into
⅜-inch-thick slices

salt and pepper to taste

nutmeg to taste

1. Heat the butter in a skillet over medium-high heat until the foam subsides. Add the zucchini and sauté for 10 minutes, stirring frequently.

2. Season with salt, pepper, and nutmeg. Serve immediately.

PER SERVING
carbs: 3 grams; Net Carbs: 2 grams;
fiber: 1 gram; protein: 1 gram; fat: 6 grams; calories: 65

PHASES 1–4

CAULIFLOWER WITH CUMIN SEED

his fragrant dish can be served either hot or at room temperature. If you are not a fan of cumin seeds, you can substitute an equal amount of fennel or caraway seeds.

PREP TIME: 10 MINUTES • COOK TIME: 10 MINUTES

4 SERVINGS

¼ cup cumin seeds

⅓ cup olive oil

4 cloves garlic, thinly sliced

1⅓ pounds cauliflower, cut into bite-size florets (4 cups)

salt and pepper to taste

1. Heat a large skillet over medium heat until hot but not smoking. Add the cumin seeds and cook for about 1 minute, until they begin to brown and pop. Remove the seeds from the skillet and reserve.

2. Add the oil to the skillet and heat over medium-high heat. Add the garlic and cook for 30 seconds. Add the cauliflower and cook, stirring occasionally, for about 5 minutes, until it begins to brown. Add the toasted cumin seeds, salt, and pepper, and toss well.

PER SERVING

carbs: 11.5 grams; Net Carbs: 7 grams;
fiber: 4.5 grams; protein: 4.5 grams; fat: 19.5 grams; calories: 223

PHASES 1–4

CAULIFLOWER—MACARONI AND CHEESE

*B*etter *than regular macaroni and cheese! Though elbow-shaped pasta is traditional, penne tastes just as good!*

PREP TIME: 10 MINUTES • COOK TIME: 25 MINUTES
6 SERVINGS

1½ cups Atkins Quick Quisine™ Pasta Cuts, penne shape

½ head cauliflower, trimmed and cut into small florets (about 2 cups)

1½ cups heavy cream

½ cup water

4 teaspoons ThickenThin™ Not Starch thickener (available at www.atkins.com)

8 ounces extra-sharp cheddar cheese, cut into small cubes

salt and pepper to taste

pinch of nutmeg

1. Cook the pasta according to package directions. Drain and rinse under cold water. Transfer to a large bowl.

2. Cook the cauliflower in lightly salted boiling water for about 5 minutes, until crisp-tender. Drain and rinse under cold water. Add to the pasta.

3. In a large saucepan, whisk together the cream, water, and thickener. Cook over medium heat for 5 minutes, whisking occasionally, until the mixture simmers and thickens. Stir in the cheese cubes, salt, pepper, and nutmeg.

4. Fold in the pasta and cauliflower. Cook, stirring gently, until heated through.

PER SERVING
carbs: 11 grams; Net Carbs: 7 grams;
fiber: 4 grams; protein: 21 grams; fat: 35 grams; calories: 420

PHASES 2–4

AVOCADO–RED PEPPER PURÉE
WITH GARLIC

This purée has a vibrant green color and creamy texture. It is a perfect accompaniment to shrimp cocktail or cold salmon. Sometimes I like to add it to mayonnaise for seafood and tuna salads. Remember this recipe when you have an avocado that has become too soft for other dishes.

PREP TIME: 10 MINUTES
MAKES ABOUT 1 CUP (8 SERVINGS)

1 ripe avocado (preferably Haas)

1 small roasted red pepper

1 small clove garlic, minced

1 tablespoon fresh lemon juice plus
    ½ teaspoon for sprinkling over
    the puree

1 tablespoon olive oil

salt and pepper to taste

2 tablespoons heavy cream

1. Halve the avocado, remove the pit, and scoop the flesh into a food processor. Add the red pepper, garlic, 1 tablespoon of lemon juice, oil, salt, and pepper. Process for 30 seconds, or until smooth. With the machine on, add the cream and process for another 15 seconds.

2. Transfer the mixture to a serving bowl and sprinkle the remaining ½ teaspoon of lemon juice on top to prevent discoloration. Serve immediately or refrigerate, in an airtight container, for up to 2 days.

PER SERVING
carbs: 2.5 grams; Net Carbs: 1.5 grams;
fiber: 1 gram; protein: 0.5 gram; fat: 7 grams; calories: 70

PHASES 1–4

ROASTED PEPPERS IN GARLIC OIL

*R*oasting peppers is really quite simple. Once the skin is charred, it pulls off easily, leaving the wonderfully sweet flesh. I sometimes chop roasted peppers and add them to chicken salad. Or bathe the roasted peppers in garlic and oil, as in this recipe, and serve them as an accompaniment to grilled fish.

PREP TIME: 10 MINUTES • COOK TIME: 10 MINUTES
4 SERVINGS

⅓ cup olive oil

2 cloves garlic, minced

2 red bell peppers

2 green bell peppers

1. Combine the oil and garlic in a bowl.

2. Roast the peppers directly over a gas flame, turning often with tongs, until the skin is completely charred, about 10 minutes. (Alternatively, roast the peppers in a preheated 450°F oven, turning frequently with tongs, until the skin is completely charred, about 20 minutes.) Transfer the peppers to a paper bag, fold the top over to seal, and set aside to steam for 10 minutes.

3. Remove the peppers from the bag. Using a small, sharp knife, scrape off all the blackened skin and remove the stem, seeds, and ribs. Cut the peppers into thin strips or coarsely chop. Add to the garlic oil and toss well. Serve immediately or refrigerate, in an airtight container, for up to 5 days.

PER SERVING
carbs: 5 grams; Net Carbs: 3.5 grams;
fiber: 1.5 grams; protein: 1 gram; fat: 18 grams; calories: 179

PHASES 1–4

VEGETABLE MEDLEY

The individual flavors of the vegetables remain distinct in this colorful medley. Serve with Garlic-Dill Meatballs (page 102).

PREP TIME: ABOUT 15 MINUTES • COOK TIME: 10 MINUTES
4 SERVINGS

---

2 tablespoons olive oil

1 small onion, finely chopped

1 yellow bell pepper, diced

1 zucchini, diced (1 cup)

½ cup peeled, seeded, and diced
    cucumber

¼ cup reduced-sodium chicken
    broth

1 clove garlic, minced

¼ teaspoon ground cumin

¼ teaspoon dried oregano

salt and pepper to taste

1. Heat the oil in a large skillet over medium-high heat until hot but not smoking. Add the onion, bell pepper, zucchini, and cucumber, and cook for 5 minutes, stirring occasionally. Add the chicken broth, garlic, cumin, oregano, salt, and pepper.

2. Bring to a boil, lower the heat, and simmer for about 10 minutes, until the vegetables are tender. Serve immediately.

PER SERVING
carbs: 4.5 grams; Net Carbs: 3.5 grams;
fiber: 1 gram; protein: 1 gram; fat: 7 grams; calories: 82

PHASES 1–4

MIXED BROILED VEGETABLES

I love making vegetable "ribbons" with a vegetable peeler. Just run a peeler lengthwise along the vegetable, and thin ribbons form. This colorful vegetable side dish is great in the summer, when basil is fresh and zucchini is abundant.

PREP TIME: 10 MINUTES • COOK TIME: 15 MINUTES
4 SERVINGS

1 small red bell pepper, cut into
   thin strips
2 tablespoons olive oil
salt and pepper to taste
1 small zucchini, sliced in ovals on
   the bias

1 small yellow squash, sliced in
   ovals on the bias
1 small carrot, cut into ribbons
   with a vegetable peeler
2 tablespoons chopped fresh basil

1. Preheat the broiler. On a jelly-roll pan, toss the bell pepper, olive oil, salt, and pepper to mix. Broil 5 inches from the heating element for 5 minutes, until the bell pepper is softened.

2. Add the zucchini, squash, and carrot to the pan, tossing to coat all the vegetables. Broil for 8 minutes, until all the vegetables are tender. Transfer to a serving bowl and toss with the basil. Serve immediately.

PER SERVING
carbs: 5.5 grams; Net Carbs: 3.5 grams;
fiber: 2 grams; protein: 1.5 grams; fat: 7 grams; calories: 85

PHASES 2–4

SAUTÉED SPINACH WITH GARLIC AND OLIVE OIL

To this classic spinach dish I have added extra garlic and the earthy hint of nutmeg. Packaged, prewashed spinach is a wonderful convenience.

PREP TIME: 5 MINUTES • COOK TIME: 5 MINUTES
4 SERVINGS

2 tablespoons olive oil

2 large cloves garlic, sliced

two 10-ounce packages washed
    baby spinach

½ chicken bouillon cube,
    crumbled

¼ teaspoon freshly grated nutmeg

salt and pepper to taste

1. Heat the olive oil in a saucepan over medium heat until hot but not smoking. Add the garlic and cook for about 1 minute, until light golden. Add the spinach and sprinkle the crumbled chicken bouillon cube on top. Partially cover the saucepan and cook, stirring from time to time, for 2–3 minutes, until the moisture has evaporated.

2. Remove the pan from the heat and stir in the nutmeg, salt, and pepper. Serve immediately.

PER SERVING
carbs: 6.5 grams; Net Carbs: 2 grams;
fiber: 4.5 grams; protein: 4.5 grams; fat: 7.5 grams; calories: 100

PHASES 1–4

CHILES RELLENOS

$\mathcal{I}$ like to add the jalapeño to these mild stuffed chilies for some kick, but they are just as delicious without it.

PREP TIME: 20 MINUTES • COOK TIME: 10 MINUTES
4 SERVINGS

6 mild California chilies
  (preferably Anaheim) or Italian
  frying peppers
⅔ cup grated Monterey Jack
  cheese
⅔ cup grated cheddar cheese

2 tablespoons seeded and chopped
  jalapeño pepper (optional)
1 large egg, lightly beaten
¼ cup Atkins Quick Quisine™
  Bake Mix or soy flour
2 tablespoons canola oil

1. Blanch the chilies in boiling salted water for 5 minutes. Rinse under cold running water. Cut open one side of the chilies and remove the stems, seeds, and ribs, keeping the chilies whole.

2. Combine the Monterey Jack, cheddar, and jalapeño, if using, in a bowl. Stuff the chilies with the cheese mixture.

3. Pour the egg onto one plate and spread the bake mix on another plate. Gently dip the chilies into the egg and then dredge them in the breading, shaking off any excess.

4. Heat the oil in a heavy skillet over medium-high heat until hot but not smoking. Add the chilies and cook, turning once, until brown, about 3 minutes per side. Serve immediately.

PER SERVING
carbs: 9 grams; Net Carbs: 6 grams;
fiber: 3 grams; protein: 16.5 grams; fat: 21 grams; calories: 285

PHASES 1−4

BROCCOLI RABE WITH
SPICY SAUSAGE

The slightly bitter taste of broccoli rabe is a perfect foil for spicy Italian sausage. The addition of balsamic vinegar adds a piquant tang. The water that clings to the broccoli rabe after it is washed should produce the right amount of liquid for cooking.

PREP TIME: 10 MINUTES • COOK TIME: 15 MINUTES
4 SERVINGS

2 tablespoons olive oil

½ pound hot Italian sausage,
    casings removed

2 cloves garlic, minced

1 pound broccoli rabe, washed

1 tablespoon balsamic vinegar

1 teaspoon freshly ground black
    pepper

½ teaspoon dried red pepper flakes

salt to taste

1. Heat the oil in a large skillet over medium-high heat until hot but not smoking. Add the sausage and cook for 6 minutes, breaking up the lumps. Add the garlic and cook for another minute.

2. Reduce the heat to low and add the broccoli rabe and vinegar (if the pan is too dry, add 1 teaspoon of water). Cover and cook, stirring occasionally, for 7 minutes, or until the broccoli rabe is tender. Stir in the black pepper, red pepper flakes, and salt. Serve immediately.

PER SERVING
carbs: 8.5 grams; Net Carbs: 2.5 grams;
fiber: 6 grams; protein: 8.5 grams; fat: 14 grams; calories: 180

PHASES 1–4

BROCCOLI PURÉE WITH GARLIC

This purée is a wonderful accompaniment to almost any entrée. For a richer dish, you can mix crème fraîche into the purée.

PREP TIME: 10 MINUTES • COOK TIME: 10 MINUTES
4 SERVINGS

2 pounds broccoli (about
   1½ heads), stems discarded
   and heads washed well and
   separated into florets

¼ cup olive oil
4 cloves garlic
salt to taste
1 teaspoon white pepper

1. Bring a large saucepan of salted water to a boil. Add the broccoli florets, cover, and cook over medium heat for 12–15 minutes, until tender. Drain.

2. In a food processor, combine the broccoli, oil, garlic, salt, and pepper. Purée until smooth, about 1 minute. Serve immediately.

PER SERVING
carbs: 8.5 grams; Net Carbs: 4 grams;
fiber: 4.5 grams; protein: 4.5 grams; fat: 14 grams; calories: 164

PHASES 1–4

GREEN BEANS WITH ANCHOVY SAUCE

*G*reen beans are a great vehicle for this salty anchovy sauce. Serve as a side dish with Grilled Lemon and Rosemary Lamb Kebobs (page 112).

PREP TIME: 10 MINUTES • COOK TIME: 5 MINUTES
4 SERVINGS

1½ pounds green beans, trimmed
  and washed
½ cup reduced-sodium chicken
  broth
3 oil-packed anchovy fillets or
  1 tablespoon homemade
  Anchovy Paste (page 159) or
  prepared anchovy paste

2 tablespoons butter
1 tablespoon chopped basil for
  garnish

1. Bring a large saucepan of salted water to a boil. Add the green beans and cook for 5 minutes.

2. While the beans are cooking, combine the broth, anchovy fillets, and butter in a small saucepan and bring to a slow boil.

3. Drain the green beans and transfer them to a bowl. Pour the anchovy sauce on top, toss well, and garnish with basil. Serve immediately.

PER SERVING
carbs: 12 grams; Net Carbs: 7 grams;
fiber: 5 grams; protein: 4 grams; fat: 6.5 grams; calories: 113

PHASES 1—4

SNOW PEAS WITH HAZELNUTS

Flavorful roasted nuts make a wonderful addition to sautéed vegetables. Hazelnuts, which are sometimes called filberts, are among my favorites.

PREP TIME: 10 MINUTES • COOK TIME: 10 MINUTES
4 SERVINGS

2 tablespoons hazelnuts, skinned
⅓ cup diced slab bacon
2 tablespoons butter

1 pound snow peas, washed
salt and pepper to taste

1. Heat a small skillet over medium heat until hot. Roast the hazelnuts, shaking the skillet occasionally, for 2–3 minutes, until golden and aromatic. Set aside.

2. Heat a large, heavy skillet over medium-high heat until hot but not smoking. Add the bacon and cook, stirring occasionally, for about 2 minutes, until browned. Using a slotted spoon, transfer the bacon to a plate. Discard the bacon fat.

3. Add the butter to the skillet and heat over low heat until the foam subsides. Add the snow peas and cook until crisp-tender, about 1 minute. Add the hazelnuts, bacon, salt, and pepper, and cook over medium-high heat, tossing gently, for 2 minutes. Serve immediately.

PER SERVING
carbs: 9 grams; Net Carbs: 5.5 grams;
fiber: 3.5 grams; protein: 5 grams; fat: 10 grams; calories: 143

PHASES 2–4

VARIATION: Substitute roasted walnuts for the hazelnuts and add 1 tablespoon of minced fresh ginger and 1 tablespoon of soy sauce to the snow peas when you add the bacon.

ASPARAGUS VINAIGRETTE

The addition of shredded radicchio really dresses up this dish for special occasions. This is great for a buffet, and using pencil asparagus eliminates the need to peel them.

PREP TIME: 10 MINUTES • COOK TIME: 10 MINUTES
4 SERVINGS

2 tablespoons chopped shallots
½ teaspoon salt
¼ teaspoon freshly ground pepper
2 tablespoons Dijon mustard
¼ cup olive oil

2½ teaspoons tarragon vinegar
2 bunches asparagus (about
   24 stalks), peeled and tied into
   2 bundles with kitchen string
1 large hard-boiled egg

1. Place the shallots in a small bowl, sprinkle with salt and pepper, and let stand for 5 minutes. Add the mustard and gradually whisk in half of the oil. Whisk in the vinegar and then the remaining oil. Cover and set aside.

2. Bring a large pot of salted water to a boil and carefully add the asparagus. Cook for 5 minutes. Transfer the asparagus to a large bowl of cold water, soak for 3 minutes, then drain.

3. Place the asparagus on a serving platter. Cut the string and discard. Drizzle the dressing evenly over the asparagus. Using a spoon, push the egg through a sieve. Sprinkle the egg over all the asparagus except the tips.

PER SERVING
carbs: 3 grams; Net Carbs: 2.5 grams;
fiber: 0.5 gram; protein: 3 grams; fat: 15.5 grams; calories: 159

PHASES 1—4

SAUTÉED KALE WITH RICOTTA SALATA

Frozen kale is just as healthy as fresh and is a great shortcut. Cooked with garlic and topped with ricotta salata (a drier version of ricotta cheese, sold in Italian delis), it is an easy and nutritious side dish. There is no need to defrost the kale before cooking.

PREP TIME: 5 MINUTES • BAKE TIME: 25 MINUTES
4 SERVINGS

1 tablespoon butter

1 tablespoon olive oil

1 clove garlic, thinly sliced

1 pound frozen kale

salt and pepper to taste

¼ cup ricotta salata

1. In a large skillet over medium-high heat, melt the butter in the olive oil. Add the garlic and cook for 1 minute, until lightly browned. Add the kale, salt, and pepper, and mix well. Cover and cook for 20 minutes, or until tender (start checking after 10 minutes, adding small amounts of water if needed).

2. Serve hot with the ricotta sprinkled on top.

PER SERVING
carbs: 6 grams; Net Carbs: 4 grams;
fiber: 2 grams; protein: 4.5 grams; fat: 9 grams; calories: 115

PHASES 2−4

SAUCES

Cucumber-Dill Sauce

Creamy Celery Sauce

Horseradish Cream

Walnut and Blue Cheese Butter

Zesty Cilantro Butter

Peanut Dipping Sauce

Caper Tartar Sauce

Creamy Mushroom Sauce

Anchovy Paste

Quick & Easy Hollandaise

Basil Pesto

CUCUMBER-DILL SAUCE

I serve this wonderfully versatile sauce with Grilled Lemon and Rosemary Lamb Kebobs (page 112) or as a burger topping. You can also whisk it with some olive oil for a quick salad dressing.

PREP TIME: 10 MINUTES

MAKES ¾ CUP

¼ cup diced cucumber

½ cup sour cream

1 teaspoon fresh lemon juice

1 tablespoon chopped fresh dill

1 teaspoon chopped fresh mint

1 small clove garlic, minced

salt and pepper to taste

Combine all the ingredients in a glass or ceramic bowl and mix well. Serve immediately or refrigerate, in an airtight container, for up to 2 days.

PER 2 TABLESPOONS

carbs: 1 gram; Net Carbs: 1 gram;

fiber: 0 grams; protein: 0.5 gram; fat: 4 grams; calories: 43

PHASES 1−4

CREAMY CELERY SAUCE

*S*erve this refreshing sauce with Beef Burgers with Feta and Tomato (page 127). It also works well as a dip for raw veggies.

PREP TIME: 5 MINUTES
MAKES ¾ CUP

—————————————— ✑ ——————————————

½ cup sour cream
¼ cup finely chopped celery
1 teaspoon ground celery seed

1 ½ teaspoons fresh lemon juice
salt and pepper to taste

Whisk together all the ingredients in a bowl. Serve immediately or refrigerate, in an airtight container, for up to 4 days.

PER 2 TABLESPOONS
carbs: 1 gram; Net Carbs: 1 gram;
fiber: 0 grams; protein: 0.5 gram; fat: 4 grams; calories: 44

PHASES 1–4

HORSERADISH CREAM

This versatile British sauce is traditionally served over thinly sliced steak. It also makes an ideal accompaniment for cold Oven-Poached Salmon with Dill and Wine (page 72).

(page 72).

PREP TIME: 5 MINUTES
MAKES ¾ CUP

⅓ cup heavy cream

1 teaspoon Dijon mustard

1½ tablespoons drained white
    horseradish

1 tablespoon sour cream

salt and pepper to taste

1. Blend the cream and mustard in a food processor or beat with an electric mixer until soft peaks form.

2. Whisk together the horseradish, sour cream, salt, and pepper until smooth.

3. Fold the mustard cream mixture into the horseradish mixture. Serve immediately or refrigerate, in an airtight container, for up to 3 days.

PER 2 TABLESPOONS
carbs: 1 gram; Net Carbs: 1 gram;
fiber: 0 grams; protein: 0.5 gram; fat: 5.5 grams; calories: 53

PHASES 1–4

WALNUT AND BLUE CHEESE BUTTER

This rich butter can turn a simple cut of beef into an elegant dish. I also like to combine it with cauliflower florets and bake the mixture for a creative alternative to the traditional "au gratin."

PREP TIME: 10 MINUTES

MAKES ½ CUP

2 ounces blue cheese, crumbled

1½ tablespoons butter, softened

1 teaspoon finely chopped fresh
flat-leaf parsley

1 teaspoon finely chopped fresh
rosemary or thyme

1 tablespoon chopped toasted
walnuts (see Hint)

Combine all the ingredients in a glass or ceramic bowl and mix well. Serve immediately or refrigerate, covered, for up to 3 days.

PER 2 TABLESPOONS
carbs: 0.5 gram; Net Carbs: 0.5 gram;
fiber: 0 grams; protein: 3.5 grams; fat: 9.5 grams; calories: 101

PHASES 2−4

HINT: To toast nuts, heat a heavy skillet over medium heat until it is hot. Cook the nuts, stirring constantly, until they become very aromatic and begin to turn brown, about 3 minutes (don't let them burn).

ZESTY CILANTRO BUTTER

Y̦ou can serve this wonderful butter on string beans or use it to sauté broccoli. Or jazz up broiled chicken by topping it with a tablespoon or two of the butter just before the chicken is finished cooking.

PREP TIME: 10 MINUTES
MAKES ¼ CUP

---

3 tablespoons butter, softened
1½ tablespoons chopped fresh
   cilantro

1½ teaspoons lemon or lime zest
1 teaspoon fresh lemon or
   lime juice

Combine all the ingredients in a bowl and mix well. Serve immediately or refrigerate, in an airtight container, for up to 1 week.

PER 1 TABLESPOON
carbs: 0 grams; Net Carbs: 0 grams;
fiber: 0 grams; protein: 0 grams; fat: 9 grams; calories: 77

PHASES 1–4

PEANUT DIPPING SAUCE

*P*eanut dipping sauce is so tasty and easy to make. Serve it with Chicken
Coconut Satay with Cilantro (page 90). You can also add a couple of tablespoons of dipping sauce to stir-fried vegetables for a distinctive Asian flavor.

PREP TIME: 10 MINUTES
MAKES 1 CUP

3 tablespoons unsweetened, non-
    hydrogenated peanut butter
1 tablespoon unsweetened coconut
    milk
1 tablespoon toasted sesame oil

½ cup water
1 tablespoon soy sauce
1 tablespoon lime juice
1 small clove garlic
½ cup coarsely chopped cilantro

Combine all the ingredients in a food processor and purée until
smooth. (If the sauce is too thick, add a bit more water.) Serve immediately
or refrigerate, covered, for up to 4 days.

PER 2 TABLESPOONS
carbs: 1.5 grams; Net Carbs: 1 gram;
fiber: 0.5 gram; protein: 2 grams; fat: 5 grams; calories: 57

PHASES 2−4

CAPER TARTAR SAUCE

*T*angy *capers give a wonderful flavor and texture to this homemade tartar sauce. I like it with a dash of hot sauce.*

PREP TIME: 5 MINUTES
MAKES ¾ CUP

½ cup mayonnaise

2 teaspoons nonpareil capers or
 chopped large capers

1 teaspoon Dijon mustard

1 teaspoon drained white
 horseradish

1½ teaspoons fresh lemon juice

1 teaspoon grated onion

salt and pepper to taste

dash of hot pepper sauce (optional)

In a bowl, whisk together all the ingredients until well blended. Serve immediately or refrigerate, in an airtight container, for up to 3 days.

PER 2 TABLESPOONS
carbs: 1 gram; Net Carbs: 1 gram;
fiber: 0 grams; protein: 0.5 gram; fat: 14.5 grams; calories: 134

PHASES 1–4

CREAMY MUSHROOM SAUCE

This versatile mushroom sauce enhances simple grilled steaks and chops, as well as Garlic-Dill Meatballs (page 102).

PREP TIME: 10 MINUTES • COOK TIME: 10 MINUTES
MAKES 1 CUP

1 tablespoon butter

½ pound button mushrooms, finely
   chopped

½ cup chicken stock

2 tablespoons heavy cream

1 tablespoon sour cream

salt and pepper to taste

nutmeg to taste

1. Heat the butter in a skillet over medium heat until the foam subsides. Add the mushrooms, and cook, stirring frequently, for 5 minutes.

2. Add the chicken stock and heavy cream and cook for 2 minutes. Remove from heat and stir in the sour cream, salt, pepper, and nutmeg. Serve immediately or refrigerate, covered, for up to 1 day.

PER 2 TABLESPOONS
carbs: 1.5 grams; Net Carbs: 1 gram;
fiber: 0.5 gram; protein: 1 gram; fat: 3.5 grams; calories: 37

PHASES 1–4

ANCHOVY PASTE

lthough anchovy paste is available ready-made, I prefer to make it myself so I can control the saltiness. I keep it on hand for whipping up Caesar Salad Dressing (page 168) and Deviled Eggs (page 13).

PREP TIME: 5 MINUTES
MAKES ¼ CUP

one 2-ounce can oil-packed
anchovies

1½ teaspoons lemon zest
1 tablespoon olive oil

1. Gently rinse the anchovies in water and pat them dry.

2. Place the anchovies, lemon zest, and oil in a food processor and purée for 20 seconds, or until smooth. Scrape down the sides and purée for another 5 seconds. (If the purée is too chunky, add a bit more oil and purée again.) Use immediately or refrigerate, in an airtight container, for up to 1 week.

PER 1 TABLESPOON
carbs: 0 grams; Net Carbs: 0 grams;
fiber: 0 grams; protein: 3 grams; fat: 4.5 grams; calories: 54

PHASES 1—4

QUICK & EASY HOLLANDAISE

This fabulously fast blender version of the classic sauce is an easy occasional treat. (If you are not comfortable eating raw eggs, skip this recipe.)

PREP TIME: 5 MINUTES • COOK TIME: 1 MINUTE
4 SERVINGS (¼ CUP PER SERVING)

⅔ cup butter

4 egg yolks

2 tablespoons fresh lemon juice

salt to taste

cayenne pepper to taste

nutmeg to taste (optional)

1. Melt the butter in a saucepan over low heat until gently bubbling.

2. Meanwhile, place the egg yolks in a blender or food processor and blend for a few seconds. With the motor running, add the lemon juice, salt, cayenne, and nutmeg. Slowly add the melted butter in a thin stream and blend for 10 seconds, or until thickened and smooth.

PER SERVING
carbs: 1 gram; Net Carbs: 1 gram;
fiber: 0 grams; protein: 3 grams; fat: 35.5 grams; calories: 330

PHASES 1−4

BASIL PESTO

*P*repared pesto from the supermarket is fine in a pinch, but for really fresh flavor, nothing beats homemade.

PREP TIME: 15 MINUTES
MAKES ¾ CUP

———— ✣ ————

2 cloves garlic

1½ cups fresh basil leaves, washed
   and dried

3 tablespoons pine nuts

3 tablespoons freshly grated
   Parmesan cheese

⅓ cup olive oil

salt and pepper to taste

1. Place the garlic, basil leaves, pine nuts, and Parmesan in a food processor and blend for a few seconds. Scrape down the sides. With the motor running, add the olive oil in a steady stream and process until puréed, about 1 minute.

2. Transfer the mixture to a bowl and mix in the salt and pepper. Serve immediately or refrigerate, covered, for up to 2 days.

PER 2 TABLESPOONS
carbs: 1.5 grams; Net Carbs: 1 gram;
fiber: 0.5 gram; protein: 2.5 grams; fat: 15 grams; calories: 145

PHASES 2−4

DRESSINGS

Quick & Easy Salad Dressing
Shallot-Orange Vinaigrette
Smoked Salmon Dressing
Caesar Salad Dressing
Creamy Italian Dressing
Asian Dressing
Poppyseed Dressing

QUICK & EASY SALAD DRESSING

*B*ottled salad dressings often contain sugar or corn syrup, which boosts the carbohydrate grams. You can make your own delicious dressing with some basic ingredients that you probably have in your pantry.

PREP TIME: 5 MINUTES
MAKES ½ CUP

2 oil-packed anchovy fillets

3 tablespoons olive oil

1½ tablespoons good-quality vinegar (such as wine, cider, or sherry)

1 tablespoon Dijon mustard

salt and pepper to taste

Mash the anchovies with a fork. Place them in a small jar that has a tight-fitting lid. Add the oil, vinegar, mustard, salt, and pepper. Cover the jar and shake vigorously until well blended, about 15–30 seconds. Serve immediately or refrigerate, covered, for up to 4 days. Shake the dressing before serving.

PER 2 TABLESPOONS
carbs: 1 gram; Net Carbs: 1 gram;
fiber: 0 grams; protein: 1 gram; fat: 10.5 grams; calories: 100

PHASES 1−4

SHALLOT-ORANGE VINAIGRETTE

This tangy, slightly sweet vinaigrette can also be used as a marinade for beef, pork, or lamb.

PREP TIME: 10 MINUTES

MAKES 1 CUP

---

2 tablespoons balsamic vinegar

2 tablespoons red wine vinegar

2 tablespoons orange juice

1 tablespoon chopped shallots

2 teaspoons Dijon mustard

1 teaspoon grated orange zest

salt and pepper to taste

¾ cup olive oil

Place the vinegars, orange juice, shallots, mustard, zest, salt, and pepper in a food processor and process until smooth. With the motor running, slowly add the olive oil until blended. Use immediately or refrigerate, in an airtight container, for up to 1 week.

PER 2 TABLESPOONS

carbs: 1.5 grams; Net Carbs: 1.5 grams;
fiber: 0 grams; protein: 0 grams; fat: 20 grams; calories: 185

PHASES 2−4

SMOKED SALMON DRESSING

This unusual dressing is great on mixed field greens. It is also delicious as an accompaniment to steamed asparagus or as a dip for crudités.

PREP TIME: 10 MINUTES

MAKES 1 CUP

¼ cup sour cream

½ cup mayonnaise

1½ ounces thinly sliced smoked
  salmon

2 teaspoons white wine vinegar

3 teaspoons fresh lemon juice

2 scallions, chopped

Combine all the ingredients in a food processor and purée for 1 minute, or until smooth. Serve immediately or refrigerate, in an airtight container, for up to 2 days.

PER 2 TABLESPOONS
carbs: 1 gram; Net Carbs: 1 gram;
fiber: 0 grams; protein: 1.5 grams; fat: 12.5 grams; calories: 123

PHASES 1–4

CAESAR SALAD DRESSING

*T**his recipe eliminates the uncooked eggs found in more traditional versions.*

PREP TIME: 5 MINUTES
MAKES ½ CUP

⁂

⅓ cup mayonnaise

2 tablespoons extra-virgin olive oil

2 tablespoons fresh lemon juice

1 clove garlic, minced

1 tablespoon Dijon mustard

2 teaspoons anchovy paste

¼ teaspoon Worcestershire sauce

salt and pepper to taste

Combine all the ingredients in a bowl and mix well. Use immediately or refrigerate, in an airtight container, for up to 3 days.

PER 2 TABLESPOONS

carbs: 2 grams; Net Carbs: 2 grams;

fiber: 0 grams; protein: 1 gram; fat: 22 grams; calories: 203

PHASES 1—4

CREAMY ITALIAN DRESSING

This homemade version is much better than store-bought and is also an excellent sauce for cold poached salmon or chicken.

PREP TIME: 10 MINUTES

MAKES 1 CUP

⅔ cup mayonnaise

¼ cup heavy cream

2 tablespoons finely chopped flat-
   leaf parsley

1 tablespoon white wine vinegar

1 garlic clove, minced

1 teaspoon dried oregano

¼ teaspoon salt

¼ teaspoon pepper

Mix the mayonnaise and cream until smooth. Add the remaining ingredients and mix well. Serve immediately or refrigerate, covered, for 3 days.

PER 2 TABLESPOONS
carbs: 0.5 gram; Net Carbs: 0.5 gram;
fiber: 0 grams; protein: 0.5 gram; fat: 17.5 grams; calories: 159

PHASES 1–4

ASIAN DRESSING

I love this dressing on any steamed or roasted green vegetable—and it is made entirely from pantry ingredients.

PREP TIME: 5 MINUTES
MAKES ¾ CUP

½ cup peanut oil

2 tablespoons sesame oil

2 tablespoons rice wine vinegar

1 tablespoon soy sauce

1 clove garlic, minced

½ packet sugar substitute

½ teaspoon hot chili paste

(optional)

Whisk together all the ingredients in a bowl. Serve immediately or refrigerate, covered, for up to 5 days.

PER 1½ TABLESPOONS
carbs: 0.5 gram; Net Carbs: 0.5 gram;
fiber: 0 grams; protein: 0 grams; fat: 17 grams; calories: 152

PHASES 1−4

POPPYSEED DRESSING

This dressing is delicious over fruit salads.

PREP TIME: 10 MINUTES

MAKES ¾ CUP

½ cup sour cream

¼ cup heavy cream

2 teaspoons poppyseeds

2 teaspoons grated lemon zest

2 packets sugar substitute

Whisk together all the ingredients until thoroughly blended. Serve immediately or refrigerate, covered, for 3 days.

PER 3 TABLESPOONS
carbs: 2.5 grams; Net Carbs: 2.5 grams,
fiber: 0 grams; protein: 1.5 grams; fat: 12 grams; calories: 122

PHASES 1−4

BREADS AND PIZZAS

Cheddar Cheese Bread

Bacon-Pepper Bread

Atkins Cornbread

Sesame–Sour Cream Muffins

Butter Rum Muffins

Savory Cheese Bites

Atkins Bread Crumbs

White Pizza with Broccoli

Veggie and Sausage Pizza

CHEDDAR CHEESE BREAD

$\mathcal{I}$nfused with mellow cheddar, this bread is rich and satisfying.

PREP TIME: 10 MINUTES • BAKE TIME: 25 MINUTES
MAKES 1 LOAF (8 SLICES)

butter for greasing the loaf pan
⅓ cup soy flour (available at
    natural-food stores)
⅓ cup whey protein (available at
    natural-food stores)

½ teaspoon baking powder
2 large eggs
2 tablespoons sour cream
2 tablespoons olive oil
½ cup grated cheddar cheese

1. Preheat the oven to 375°F. Generously butter an 8 × 4-inch loaf pan.

2. In a bowl, combine the soy flour, whey, and baking powder. Stir in the eggs, sour cream, and olive oil and mix well. Fold in half of the cheddar.

3. Pour the batter into the prepared pan and sprinkle the remaining cheddar on top. Bake for 25 minutes, or until a cake tester comes out clean. Serve immediately or let it cool, then wrap well in plastic wrap and refrigerate for up to 2 days or freeze for up to 1 month.

PER SLICE
carbs: 5 grams; Net Carbs: 4.5 grams;
fiber: 0.5 gram; protein: 5 grams; fat: 8.5 grams; calories: 118

PHASES 1−4

BACON-PEPPER BREAD

*S*erve this flavorful bread with eggs for breakfast or with egg salad on a bed
of lettuce for a light lunch.

PREP TIME: 15 MINUTES • BAKE TIME: 25 MINUTES
MAKES 1 LOAF (8 SLICES)

butter for greasing the loaf pan

⅓ cup soy flour (available at
    natural-food stores)

⅓ cup whey protein (available at
    natural-food stores)

½ teaspoon baking powder

2 large eggs

2 tablespoons sour cream

½ teaspoon freshly ground pepper

3 slices bacon, cooked and
    crumbled

1. Preheat the oven to 375°F. Generously butter an 8 × 4-inch
loaf pan.

2. In a bowl, combine the soy flour, whey, and baking powder. Stir in the
eggs, sour cream, and pepper and mix well. Fold in half of the bacon bits.

3. Pour the batter into the prepared pan and sprinkle the remaining
bacon on top. Bake for 25 minutes, or until a cake tester comes out clean.
Serve immediately or let cool, then wrap well in plastic wrap and refrigerate for up to 2 days or freeze for up to 1 month.

PER SLICE
carbs: 5.5 grams; Net Carbs: 5 grams;
fiber: 0.5 gram; protein: 4 grams; fat: 4 grams; calories: 74

PHASES 1−4

ATKINS CORNBREAD

*T*his *"cornbread" contains no cornmeal, but it is a perfect accompaniment for fried chicken or a bowl of stew. Wheat gluten gives the bread its distinctive chewiness.*

PREP TIME: 10 MINUTES • COOK TIME: 35 MINUTES
9 SERVINGS

½ cup Atkins Quick Quisine™
  Bake Mix

¼ cup wheat gluten (available at
  natural-food stores)

3 eggs

1 cup milk

4 ounces jalapeño Jack cheese,
  grated

1 chipotle en adobo, finely chopped
  (optional)

⅓ cup vegetable oil

1. Preheat the oven to 450°F. Whisk together the bake mix, gluten, eggs, and milk. Fold in the grated cheese and chipotle, if using.

2. Pour the oil into an 8-inch square baking pan and place it on the middle rack of the oven. Heat for 10 minutes, until very hot. Pour the batter in and bake for 15 minutes.

3. Lower the temperature to 350°F and cook for 20 minutes more, until browned on top. Cool the bread on a wire rack before cutting into 9 squares.

PER SERVING
carbs: 5 grams; Net Carbs: 4.5 grams;
fiber: 0.5 gram; protein: 8 grams; fat: 15 grams; calories: 201

PHASES 1–4

SESAME–SOUR CREAM MUFFINS

*Y*ou choose: Spread butter, cream cheese, or pâté on these savory muffins. *They make a great accompaniment for soup or a salad.*

PREP TIME: 10 MINUTES • BAKE TIME: 25 MINUTES
MAKES 6 MUFFINS

butter for greasing the muffin pans
¼ cup soy flour (available at
   natural-food stores)
¼ cup ground sesame seeds
   (available at natural-food stores)

2 eggs
3 tablespoons sour cream
2 tablespoons butter, melted
½ teaspoon baking powder

1. Preheat the oven to 350°F. Generously butter six ½-cup muffin pans.

2. Combine all the ingredients in a food processor and process for 2–3 minutes or until smooth.

3. Divide the batter evenly among the muffin pans, filling each about three-fourths full. Bake for 20–25 minutes, or until a cake tester comes out clean.

4. Let the muffins sit in the pans for 5 minutes, then turn them out onto a wire rack to cool completely.

PER SERVING
carbs: 2.5 grams; Net Carbs: 1.5 grams;
fiber: 1 gram; protein: 5 grams; fat: 10.5 grams; calories: 124

PHASES 2–4

BUTTER RUM MUFFINS

These fragrant muffins will make any breakfast special. They are great for afternoon tea, too. For luscious homemade blueberry muffins, add ¼ cup blueberries to the batter.

PREP TIME: 15 MINUTES • BAKE TIME: 25 MINUTES
MAKES 4 MUFFINS

butter for greasing the muffin pans

¼ cup soy flour (available at natural-food stores)

¼ cup ground sesame seeds (available at natural-food stores)

¼ teaspoon whey protein (available at natural-food stores)

2 large eggs

3 tablespoons sour cream

1 tablespoon butter, softened

1 teaspoon rum

1½ packets sugar substitute

½ teaspoon vanilla extract

½ teaspoon baking powder

1. Preheat the oven to 350°F. Generously butter six ½-cup muffin pans.

2. Combine all the ingredients in a food processor and process for 2–3 minutes or until smooth.

3. Divide the batter evenly among the muffin pans, filling each about three-fourths full. Bake for 20–25 minutes, or until a cake tester comes out clean.

4. Let the muffins sit in the pans for 5 minutes, then turn them out onto a wire rack to cool completely.

PER SERVING
carbs: 10 grams; Net Carbs: 8.5 grams;
fiber: 1.5 grams; protein: 8 grams; fat: 13 grams; calories: 193

PHASES 2–4

SAVORY CHEESE BITES

*T*hese appetizing crackers have a cookielike texture. Serve them with soups and salads.

PREP TIME: 10 MINUTES • BAKE TIME: 18 MINUTES
6 SERVINGS

cooking spray (see Note)

¾ cup Atkins Quick Quisine™
   Bake Mix

4 tablespoons butter

2 egg whites

¼ cup sunflower seeds

⅓ cup grated Parmesan cheese

1 tablespoon lemon juice

1 tablespoon grated lemon zest

¼ teaspoon salt

½ teaspoon pepper

⅓ cup seltzer

1. Preheat the oven to 375°F. Coat a baking sheet with cooking spray.

2. In a bowl, thoroughly mix all the ingredients.

3. Drop heaping tablespoons of batter onto the baking sheet. Bake for 18 minutes, or until lightly golden. Cool on the baking sheet for 5 minutes, then transfer the "bites" to a wire rack to cool completely. Serve immediately, or store in an airtight container for up to 3 days.

PER SERVING
carbs: 4.5 grams; Net Carbs: 2.5 grams;
fiber: 2 grams; protein: 13.5 grams; fat: 14.5 grams; calories: 201

PHASES 2–4

NOTE: To make your own cooking spray, fill a small spray bottle with canola oil.

ATKINS BREAD CRUMBS

*F*or breading cutlets, binding meatballs and stuffing, and making fried snacks, flavored bread crumbs are a must-have item. Whip up a batch and freeze to have on hand anytime.

PREP TIME: 5 MINUTES • COOK TIME: 15 MINUTES
6 SERVINGS

5 slices Atkins Bakery™ Ready-to-Eat Sliced White or Rye Bread, frozen

¼ cup grated Parmesan cheese

1 teaspoon Italian seasoning (or a mix of oregano, basil, and parsley)

¼ teaspoon kosher salt

¼ teaspoon pepper

1. Preheat the oven to 350°F.

2. Cut the frozen bread into 1-inch cubes. Spread them in a single layer on a baking sheet. Bake for 15 minutes, until thoroughly dry but not brown.

3. In a food processor, process the cubes into fine crumbs. Add the Parmesan, Italian seasoning, salt, and pepper. Pulse to combine.

PER SERVING
carbs: 8 grams; Net Carbs: 3 grams;
fiber: 5 grams; protein: 8 grams; fat: 1.5 grams; calories: 69

PHASES 1–4

WHITE PIZZA WITH BROCCOLI

$\mathcal{T}$*he actual work time in this recipe is short, and you can do other things while the pizza dough rises. This was a favorite of Dr. Atkins.*

PREP TIME: 30 MINUTES • COOK TIME: 20 MINUTES
RISING TIME: 1 HOUR
8 SERVINGS

---

1 box (12.6 oz.) Atkins Quick &
  Easy™ Country White Bread
  Mix
5 tablespoons extra-virgin olive oil
2 cloves garlic, minced
2 cups cooked broccoli florets

¾ cup whole-milk ricotta cheese
½ cup shredded mozzarella cheese
2 tablespoons grated Parmesan
  cheese
½ teaspoon dried oregano

1. Combine the bread mix and included yeast in a large bowl. Add 1½ cups warm water and 3 tablespoons olive oil. Mix with a spoon to form a soft dough. Knead gently for 1 minute. Shape the dough into a ball, cover with plastic wrap, and let rise for 1 hour, or until the dough is doubled in size.

2. While the dough is rising, heat 1 tablespoon of the oil in a large skillet over medium heat. Cook the garlic for 30 seconds, until starting to color. Add the broccoli and cook for 2 minutes, until heated through. Remove the skillet from the heat and stir in the ricotta.

3. Preheat the oven to 450°F.

4. Shape the pizza dough into a 14-inch round and transfer it to a wire mesh pizza screen or a pizza pan with holes. Spread the broccoli mixture over the dough, leaving a ½-inch border. Top with the mozzarella and Parmesan. Sprinkle with the oregano and remaining 1 tablespoon of oil.

5. Bake the pizza for 20–22 minutes, or until puffed and nicely browned. Serve immediately.

PER SERVING
carbs: 18.5 grams; Net Carbs: 7.5 grams;
fiber: 11 grams; protein: 29 grams; fat: 13.5 grams; calories: 285

PHASES 2–4

VEGGIE AND SAUSAGE PIZZA

*I*f you are not partial to the distinctive flavor of goat cheese, substitute cheddar or mozzarella.

PREP TIME: 30 MINUTES • COOK TIME: 20 MINUTES

RISING TIME: 1 HOUR

8 SERVINGS

1 box (12.6 oz.) Atkins Quick & Easy™ Country White Bread Mix

5 tablespoons extra-virgin olive oil

½ medium eggplant, cut into ¼-inch slices

1 teaspoon salt

1 cup low carb tomato sauce

1 cup cooked crumbled Italian sausage (about 4 links)

½ small bell pepper, thinly sliced

2 ounces goat cheese, crumbled

¼ cup fresh basil leaves, chopped

1. Combine the bread mix and included yeast in a large bowl. Add 1½ cups warm water and 3 tablespoons olive oil. Mix with a spoon to form a soft dough. Knead the dough gently for 1 minute. Shape it into a ball, cover with plastic wrap, and let rise for 1 hour, or until the dough is doubled in size.

2. While the dough is rising, sprinkle the eggplant with salt and place it in a colander to drain for 30 minutes. Rinse and pat dry.

3. Preheat the oven to 450°F. Brush the eggplant slices with the remaining 2 tablespoons of olive oil and place in a single layer on a nonstick baking sheet. Bake for 10 minutes, turning once.

4. Shape the dough into a 14-inch round and transfer it to a wire mesh pizza screen or a pizza pan with holes. Spread the tomato sauce on the dough, leaving a ½-inch border. Top with the eggplant, sausage, pepper, and goat cheese. Spread the toppings as close to the edge as possible.

5. Bake the pizza for 20–22 minutes, or until puffed and browned. Remove from the oven and sprinkle with the basil. Serve immediately.

PER SERVING

carbs: 20 grams; Net Carbs: 9 grams;

fiber: 11 grams; protein: 29 grams; fat: 15.5 grams; calories: 311

PHASES 2–4

DESSERTS

Chocolate Buttercream
Shortcakes Véronique with a Kiss of Rum
Hazelnut Torte
Strawberry Shortcakes
Lemon-Poppy Pound Cake
Coconut Custard Pudding
Zabaglione
Vanilla and Raspberry Parfaits
Cranberry-Hazelnut Biscotti
Cookie Cutouts
Berries with Chocolate Ganache
Broiled Pineapple with Ice Cream and Almonds

CHOCOLATE BUTTERCREAM

This velvety chocolate cream tastes wonderful either on its own or with the Hazelnut Torte (page 189).

PREP TIME: 5 MINUTES • COOK TIME: 7 MINUTES
MAKES 1 CUP

4 egg yolks

2 tablespoons cognac

½ teaspoon vanilla extract

2 tablespoons finely chopped
    unsweetened dark chocolate

4 packets sugar substitute

8 tablespoons unsalted butter,
    softened

1. Beat all the ingredients in a large bowl with an electric mixer for 2 minutes.

2. Place the mixture in the top of a double boiler over gently simmering water and cook, stirring constantly, for 7 minutes. Remove from the heat and serve immediately.

PER 2 TABLESPOONS
carbs: 1 gram; Net Carbs: 1 gram;
fiber: 0 grams; protein: 1.5 grams; fat: 15 grams; calories: 153

PHASES 1–4

Shortcakes Véronique
with a Kiss of Rum

*N*o one will believe that this dessert can be part of a controlled carb program! The rum adds a depth of flavor that is perfectly complemented by the
fresh berries.

PREP TIME: 10 MINUTES
4 SERVINGS

4 Butter Rum Muffins (page 179),
  halved
4 teaspoons rum (do not substitute
  liqueurs, which are high in
  sugar)
½ cup heavy cream

1 packet sugar substitute
¼ cup blueberries or raspberries (or
  a combination)
4 large strawberries, halved
4 mint sprigs for garnish (optional)

1. Sprinkle the muffin halves with rum.
2. With an electric mixer on medium, beat the cream and sugar substitute until soft peaks form.
3. Spread the whipped cream over the muffin halves and top with the
berries.
4. Place 2 shortcake halves on each plate. Place a mint sprig between
the halves.

PER SERVING
carbs: 13.5 grams; Net Carbs: 11.5 grams;
fiber: 2 grams; protein: 9 grams; fat: 24 grams; calories: 318

PHASES 3 AND 4

HAZELNUT TORTE

This baked hazelnut torte has a rich flavor and a wonderful aroma. Serve with whipped cream or Chocolate Buttercream (page 187).

PREP TIME: 10 MINUTES • BAKE TIME: 25 MINUTES
4 SERVINGS

¾ cup plus 2 tablespoons ground
   hazelnuts, divided
1 tablespoon whey protein
   (available at natural-food stores)
3 packets sugar substitute

½ tablespoon baking powder
2 eggs
1 tablespoon sour cream
butter for greasing the cake pan

1. Preheat the oven to 350°F. In a large bowl, combine ¾ cup plus 1 tablespoon hazelnuts, whey, sugar substitute, and baking powder. Using an electric mixer, mix in the eggs and sour cream on medium-high speed for about 2 minutes, until fluffy.

2. Generously butter an 8-inch round cake pan and sprinkle the remaining 1 tablespoon of hazelnuts over the bottom of the pan. Scrape in the cake batter and smooth the top.

3. Bake for 25 minutes, or until a cake tester comes out clean. Cool in the pan for 10 minutes, then invert onto a wire rack to cool completely. Cut into quarters, and serve.

PER SERVING
carbs: 5.5 grams; Net Carbs: 4 grams;
fiber: 1.5 grams; protein: 6 grams; fat: 13.5 grams; calories: 159

PHASES 2−4

STRAWBERRY SHORTCAKES

This is a wonderful summer dessert, when strawberries are at their peak. Delicious as they are, these shortcakes are even better when topped with whipped cream sweetened with sugar substitute.

PREP TIME: 10 MINUTES • BAKE TIME: 20 MINUTES
4 SERVINGS

1 cup Atkins Quick Quisine™
    Bake Mix
1 teaspoon baking powder
¼ teaspoon salt
1 tablespoon granular sugar
    substitute

2 tablespoons unsalted butter
½ cup heavy cream
½ cup water
2 cups washed, hulled strawberries,
    sliced and sweetened to taste
    with sugar substitute

1. Preheat the oven to 400°F. In a medium bowl, combine the bake mix, baking powder, salt, and sugar substitute. Cut the butter into the dry mixture with a pastry blender or two knives, until the mixture resembles coarse meal. Add the cream and water and mix to form a dough.

2. Divide the dough into 4 equal pieces and form into balls. Place the dough balls on an ungreased baking sheet and flatten slightly. Bake for 20 minutes, or until golden brown. Cool to room temperature.

3. Slice the shortcakes in half horizontally. Spoon ¼ cup of the strawberries on each bottom half, cover with the remaining halves, and top each with ¼ cup of strawberries.

PER SERVING
carbs: 12.5 grams; Net Carbs: 8 grams;
fiber: 4.5 grams; protein: 19 grams; fat: 20.5 grams; calories: 298

PHASES 2–4

LEMON-POPPY POUND CAKE

Turn delicious Atkins Quick Quisine™ Lemon Poppy Bake Mix into a pound cake by using heavy cream for added richness. A topping of strawberries and whipped cream makes this a complete dessert.

PREP TIME: 10 MINUTES • COOK TIME: 1 HOUR
12 SERVINGS

one 12-ounce box Atkins Quick Quisine™ Lemon Poppy Bake Mix

1 pint heavy cream

2 packets sugar substitute

1 quart fresh strawberries, hulled and sliced

8 tablespoons lightly toasted sliced almonds

1. Make the cake according to package directions for bread, except substitute ½ cup of heavy cream for ½ cup of the water (adding the remaining water as well). Bake as directed. Cool completely and cut into 18 slices (you will use only 12 slices for this recipe; freeze the rest).

2. Whip the remaining 1½ cups heavy cream on medium high, adding the sugar substitute, until soft peaks form.

3. Top each slice of cake with ¼ cup of berries, 2 tablespoons of whipped cream, and 2 teaspoons of almonds.

PER SERVING
carbs: 16 grams; Net Carbs: 8.5 grams;
fiber: 7.5 grams; protein: 15 grams; fat: 18 grams; calories: 265

PHASES 3 AND 4

COCONUT CUSTARD PUDDING

*R*ich and creamy, this coconut pudding has delicious butterscotch undertones.

PREP TIME: 5 MINUTES • COOK TIME: 15 MINUTES
4 SERVINGS

1 can (14 ounces) unsweetened
   coconut milk
½ cup heavy cream
3 egg yolks

1 tablespoon butterscotch extract
   or 1 teaspoon coconut extract
3 packets sugar substitute

1. Combine the coconut milk and heavy cream in a saucepan. Bring to a boil, then reduce the heat to very low.

2. Meanwhile, whisk together the egg yolks, butterscotch extract, and sugar substitute in a bowl.

3. Stirring constantly, add the egg mixture to the cream mixture, a little at a time, until incorporated. Simmer over very low heat, stirring constantly, for 5 minutes. Transfer the saucepan to a large bowl or sink filled with cold water to cool for 5 minutes. Serve at room temperature or chilled.

PER SERVING
carbs: 5 grams; Net Carbs: 4 grams;
fiber: 1 gram; protein: 4.5 grams; fat: 36 grams; calories: 355

PHASES 1−4

ZABAGLIONE

This luxurious custard is fused with rich marsala and complemented by fresh berries. It is the perfect ending for a dinner or a brunch. Enjoy!

PREP TIME: 5 MINUTES • COOK TIME: ABOUT 5 MINUTES
4 SERVINGS

8 egg yolks

3 packets sugar substitute

½ cup dry marsala

4 large ripe strawberries

½ cup blueberries

1. Combine the egg yolks, sugar substitute, and marsala in a food processor and process at high speed for about 15 seconds (don't over-blend).

2. Pour the mixture into a double boiler and simmer gently over low heat, whisking constantly, for about 5 minutes, until the mixture thickens to the consistency of whipped cream. (The custard can be refrigerated for up to two days; emulsify in a blender if it has separated.)

3. Slice the strawberries lengthwise to the stem but keep attached at the stem end. Divide the blueberries among 4 small bowls or ramekins. Pour the zabaglione on top. Fan out a strawberry and place on top of each serving. Serve immediately.

PER SERVING
carbs: 8.5 grams; Net Carbs: 7.5 grams;
fiber: 1 gram; protein: 3 grams; fat: 5 grams; calories: 123

PHASES 2−4

VANILLA AND RASPBERRY PARFAITS

These parfaits look so elegant that guests will never guess how easy they are to make.

PREP TIME: 15 MINUTES • COOK TIME: 5 MINUTES
CHILL TIME: 20 MINUTES
4 SERVINGS

1 cup heavy cream, divided
½ cup water
½ cup granular sugar substitute
dash of salt
1 egg, lightly beaten
1 teaspoon vanilla extract

2 teaspoons ThickenThin™ Not
   Starch thickener (available at
   www.atkins.com)
2 cups raspberries, rinsed
4 sprigs fresh mint

1. In a small saucepan, mix ½ cup of heavy cream and the water. Over medium heat, bring the mixture to a boil, then remove from the heat.

2. In the top of a double boiler, over medium-low heat, combine the sugar substitute, salt, and egg. Gradually whisk in the cream mixture and the vanilla. Cook for 5 minutes, stirring constantly, until the mixture coats the back of a spoon. Remove from the heat and whisk in the thickener. Refrigerate for 20 minutes.

3. Meanwhile, with an electric mixer on medium, beat the remaining ½ cup of heavy cream until soft peaks form. Stir ¼ of the whipped cream into the cooled pudding, then fold in the remaining whipped cream.

4. Assemble the parfaits in clear stemmed glasses—large wineglasses work well. Layer ¼ cup pudding and ¼ cup berries; repeat. Top each with a sprig of fresh mint and serve immediately.

PER SERVING
carbs: 12 grams; Net Carbs: 8 grams;
fiber: 4 grams; protein: 3.5 grams; fat: 23.5 grams; calories: 266

PHASES 2–4

CRANBERRY-HAZELNUT BISCOTTI

*H*azelnuts are a favorite nut in Europe. The cranberries are an American touch, making this a truly international cookie!

PREP TIME: 25 MINUTES • BAKE TIME: 40 MINUTES

MAKES 40 COOKIES

1½ cups toasted and skinned
  hazelnuts: ½ cup finely
  chopped, 1 cup coarsely
  chopped
1 cup Atkins Quick Quisine™
  Bake Mix
16 packets sugar substitute

1 teaspoon ground cinnamon
¼ teaspoon salt
¼ cup sour cream
4 eggs, lightly beaten
1½ sticks butter, at room
  temperature
⅓ cup dried cranberries

1. Preheat the oven to 350°F. Whisk together the finely chopped hazelnuts, bake mix, sugar substitute, cinnamon, and salt.

2. In a medium bowl, mix the sour cream and eggs.

3. In a large bowl, using an electric mixer on medium speed, beat the butter for 3 minutes, until creamy. In alternating batches, add the dry mixture and sour cream mixture to the butter. Stir in the cranberries and coarsely chopped hazelnuts.

4. Divide the dough in half. On ungreased baking sheets, form each dough half into a log measuring 12 inches by 2½ inches (moisten your hands if necessary to keep the dough from sticking).

5. Bake the logs for 25 minutes, until almost firm. Transfer the sheets to a wire rack to cool for 10 minutes. Reduce the oven temperature to 325°F.

6. Using a serrated knife, carefully cut the logs crosswise into ½-inch-wide slices. Arrange the slices on the baking sheets. Bake for 15–17 minutes, until firm and crisp. Cool the biscotti on the baking sheets before storing in an airtight container.

PER BISCOTTO
carbs: 2.5 grams; Net Carbs: 1.5 grams;
fiber: 1 gram; protein: 1.5 grams; fat: 7.5 grams; calories: 89

PHASES 2–4

COOKIE CUTOUTS

This is a basic cookie recipe and my favorite to bake during the holidays. The finished cookies can be glazed with sugar-free jam or sprinkled with extra sugar substitute.

PREP TIME: 20 MINUTES • CHILL TIME: 10 MINUTES
BAKE TIME: 12 MINUTES
MAKES 20 COOKIES

---

1 cup Atkins Quick Quisine™ Bake Mix plus extra for cookie cutters

3 tablespoons granular sugar substitute

4 ounces cream cheese

2 tablespoons butter

2 tablespoons sour cream

1 egg white

1 teaspoon vanilla extract

1. Preheat the oven to 350°F. Position a rack in the center of the oven.

2. Combine the bake mix, sugar substitute, cream cheese, and butter with a pastry blender. Mix together the sour cream, egg white, and vanilla extract. Add the bake mix mixture to the sour cream mixture and combine thoroughly.

3. Roll out the dough between two sheets of plastic wrap until it is ¼ inch thick. Place the dough in the freezer for 10 minutes, or until firm.

4. Remove the top layer of the plastic wrap. As you cut out cookies into desired shapes, dip the cookie cutters into the extra bake mix before each use. Arrange the cookies on a baking sheet. Bake for 11–12 minutes, until light gold and set. Cool the cookies on the baking sheet placed on a wire rack.

PER COOKIE
carbs: 1.5 grams; Net Carbs: 1 gram;
fiber: 0.5 gram; protein: 4 grams; fat: 4 grams; calories: 58

PHASES 1–4

BERRIES WITH CHOCOLATE GANACHE

A ganache is essentially a mixture of chocolate and cream, and it is one of the most delicious and easiest dessert sauces to prepare. In this recipe, I pour it over fresh berries.

PREP TIME: 10 MINUTES • COOK TIME: 5 MINUTES
4 SERVINGS

1½ Atkins Endulge™ Chocolate
    Candy Bars, broken in pieces
¼ cup heavy cream
½ teaspoon vanilla extract

1 pint strawberries, rinsed and
    halved
½ cup raspberries, rinsed
½ cup blueberries, rinsed

1. In a double boiler, melt the bars with the cream, stirring until smooth. Mix in the vanilla extract. Cool slightly.

2. Mix the berries and divide among 4 dessert dishes. Drizzle the ganache over the fruit.

PER SERVING
carbs: 11.5 grams; Net Carbs: 7 grams;
fiber: 4.5 grams; protein: 1.5 grams; fat: 10.5 grams; calories: 148

PHASES 2−4

Broiled Pineapple with Ice Cream and Almonds

$\mathcal{W}$hen you are in the mood for a quick and simple tasty dessert, this is an ideal choice.

PREP TIME: 10 MINUTES • COOK TIME: 10 MINUTES
4 SERVINGS

½ medium ripe pineapple, peeled
   and cored
4 tablespoons unsalted butter
4 tablespoons granular sugar
   substitute

1 teaspoon ground cinnamon
4 cups Atkins Endulge™ Premium
   Ice Cream Cups, vanilla flavor
2 tablespoons chopped toasted
   almonds

1. Preheat the broiler. Cut the pineapple into 1-inch-thick slices.

2. In a small saucepan or microwave-safe bowl, melt the butter. Mix in the sugar substitute and cinnamon. Brush the pineapple rings with the mixture.

3. Broil the pineapple for 5–7 minutes per side, until nicely browned. Top each serving with ½ cup ice cream and ½ tablespoon almonds.

PER SERVING
carbs: 15.5 grams; Net Carbs: 14.5 grams;
fiber: 1 gram; protein: 4 grams; fat: 27.5 grams; calories: 318

PHASES 3 AND 4

BEVERAGES

Ultrarich Strawberry Shake
Chocolate-Raspberry Smoothie
Mixed Berry Smoothie
Peach-Orange Ginger Tea
Honeydew-Lime Slushy with Mint
Lime-Raspberry Cooler
Hot Mocha with Almond Cream

ULTRARICH STRAWBERRY SHAKE

*W*hen I have no time in the morning but want to start the day right, I whip up this shake. It is a delicious way to start the day.

PREP TIME: 5 MINUTES

4 SERVINGS

12 whole strawberries

1 cup Atkins Advantage™
   Strawberry Shake Mix

1 cup heavy cream

2 teaspoons vanilla extract

4 cups cold water

4 packets sugar substitute

Place all the ingredients in a blender and blend at high speed until very smooth.

PER SERVING

carbs: 5.5 grams; Net Carbs: 4.5 grams;
fiber: 1 gram; protein: 13.5 grams; fat: 26 grams; calories: 304

PHASES 2–4

CHOCOLATE-RASPBERRY SMOOTHIE

This decadent-tasting drink has just the right balance of fruit and chocolate in a classic flavor combination.

PREP TIME: 10 MINUTES
6 SERVINGS

4 Atkins Endulge™ Premium Ice
   Cream Cups, chocolate flavor
1½ cups frozen unsweetened
   raspberries

1½ cups water
¼ cup unsweetened cocoa powder

Remove the ice cream from the cups and place it in the blender with the rest of the ingredients. Purée until smooth and thick. Scrape the sides of the blender and stir with a spatula to make sure the cocoa is well incorporated and the thickness is uniform. Purée again, if needed.

PER SERVING
carbs: 22.5 grams; Net Carbs: 18.5 grams;
fiber: 4 grams; protein: 3 grams; fat: 8 grams; calories: 158

PHASES 3 AND 4

MIXED BERRY SMOOTHIE

If you cannot find mixed frozen berries at your grocery store, use the frozen berry of your choice. Tofu adds protein and texture to this smoothie.

PREP TIME: 5 MINUTES

4 SERVINGS

---

2 berry-flavored tea bags
¾ cup boiling water
¾ cup light cranberry juice
    (see Note)
1 cup frozen unsweetened mixed
    berries

1 pound silken tofu
½ cup heavy cream
1 to 2 packets sugar substitute

1. Place the tea bags in a heatproof bowl. Add the boiling water and let steep for 4–6 minutes. Press the liquid from the tea bags before removing from the bowl. Let cool.

2. In a blender, purée the tea, cranberry juice, berries, tofu, heavy cream, and sugar substitute until smooth, scraping down the sides of the blender as needed.

PER SERVING
carbs: 13.5 grams; Net Carbs: 12.5 grams;
fiber: 1 gram; protein: 9 grams; fat: 14 grams; calories: 211

PHASES 3 AND 4

NOTE: Light cranberry juice is sweetened with Splenda®.

PEACH-ORANGE GINGER TEA

If you do not have fresh ginger, you can substitute powdered ginger. Add the powdered ginger ⅛ teaspoon at a time, tasting as you go along.

PREP TIME: 5 MINUTES • COOK TIME: 5 MINUTES
4 SERVINGS

4 bags peach tea

2-inch-square ginger knob, thinly sliced

2 tablespoons plus 2 teaspoons granular sugar substitute

1 cup boiling water

3 cups mandarin orange–flavored seltzer

1. Place the tea bags, ginger, and sugar substitute in a heatproof serving pitcher. Pour in the boiling water and let the ingredients steep for 4–6 minutes. Press the liquid from the tea bags before removing from the pitcher. Remove the ginger slices.

2. Let the tea cool to room temperature, then add the seltzer. Serve in tall glasses.

PER SERVING
carbs: 0.5 gram; Net Carbs: 0.5 gram;
fiber: 0 grams; protein: 0 grams; fat: 0 grams; calories: 0

PHASES 1–4

Honeydew-Lime Slushy with Mint

Refreshing, bracing, and icy! This versatile slushy can also double as a summertime dessert.

PREP TIME: 10 MINUTES

4 SERVINGS

———————————— ✍ ————————————

3 cups honeydew melon cubes

2 cups ice cubes

¼ cup fresh mint leaves plus extra
  for garnish

¼ cup lime juice

2 teaspoons grated lime zest

Combine half of the honeydew, ice, mint, lime juice, and zest in a blender. Purée until slushy. Pour into two tall glasses. Repeat with remaining half of ingredients. Garnish with mint sprigs and serve immediately.

PER SERVING
carbs: 13.5 grams; Net Carbs: 12.5 grams;
fiber: 1 gram; protein: 1 gram; fat: 0 grams; calories: 51

PHASES 3 AND 4

LIME-RASPBERRY COOLER

This drink allows you to enjoy fruit flavors even on Induction. For a pretty presentation, garnish each glass with a thin slice of lime.

PREP TIME: 5 MINUTES
4 SERVINGS

4 bags Red Zinger tea

2 tablespoons granular sugar
   substitute

2 tablespoons lime juice

2 teaspoons grated lime zest

2 cups boiling water

2 cups raspberry-flavored seltzer

1. Place the tea bags, sugar substitute, lime juice, and zest in a heat-proof serving pitcher. Pour the boiling water into the pitcher and let steep for 4–6 minutes. Press the liquid from the tea bags before removing from the pitcher.

2. Cool the tea to room temperature, then add the seltzer. Pour through a strainer into tall glasses.

PER SERVING
carbs: 1 gram; Net Carbs: 1 gram;
fiber: 0 grams; protein: 0 grams; fat: 0 grams; calories: 3

PHASES 1–4

HOT MOCHA WITH ALMOND CREAM

T̶his warm, soothing drink is even more heavenly if you replace some of the water with heavy cream, which will increase the carb count.

PREP TIME: 5 MINUTES • COOK TIME: 5 MINUTES
4 SERVINGS

1 tablespoon plus 1 teaspoon
  instant decaffeinated coffee

⅛ teaspoon salt

5 tablespoons unsweetened cocoa
  powder

⅓ cup granular sugar substitute,
  divided

4 cups boiling water, divided

½ cup heavy cream

¼ teaspoon almond extract

¼ teaspoon vanilla extract

1. In a pitcher, whisk together the coffee, salt, cocoa, and all but 1 tablespoon of the sugar substitute. Slowly whisk in 1 cup of boiling water until a smooth paste forms. Pour in the remaining 3 cups of boiling water and mix well. Pour into coffee mugs.

2. In a bowl, combine the cream, almond and vanilla extracts, and remaining 1 tablespoon of sugar substitute. Whisk vigorously until soft peaks form. Top each coffee with a dollop of almond cream.

PER SERVING
carbs: 6 grams; Net Carbs: 4 grams;
fiber: 2 grams; protein: 2 grams; fat: 12 grams; calories: 124

PHASES 1−4

ACCEPTABLE FOODS

The premise of the four phases of the Atkins Nutritional Approach™ is twofold. First, you cut back on all carbs and reduce your intake to 20 grams of Net Carbs a day to kick-start weight loss in Induction. In that phase, your carbohydrates come primarily from salad greens and other low-glycemic vegetables. Then, as you proceed to Ongoing Weight Loss after a minimum of two weeks, you gradually add both grams of carbohydrate and reintroduce other carbohydrate foods. By the time you reach Lifetime Maintenance, you should have reintroduced almost all carbohydrate foods with the exception of sugar, bleached flour, and processed foods. You will have also raised your carbohydrate intake to as many grams of Net Carbs as you can eat without regaining weight.

Note: Not everyone is able to reintroduce all foods into his or her diet without regaining weight.

Acceptable Foods During the Induction Phase

PROTEIN
You can eat liberal amounts of the following foods, meaning you should eat until you are satisfyingly full but not stuffed.

MEAT
Beef
Lamb
Pork/Ham/Bacon

Rabbit
Veal
Venison

Note: Processed meats such as bacon, ham, pepperoni, salami, hot dogs, and other luncheon meats, and even some fish, may be cured with added sugar, which can up your carb count. Also avoid luncheon meats with nitrates. Do not consume more than 4 ounces of organ meats (such as liver) a day. Avoid products that are not exclusively meat (or fish or fowl), such as meat loaf or breaded foods.

POULTRY
Chicken
Cornish hen
Duck
Goose
Pheasant
Quail (and other game birds)
Turkey

FISH (INCLUDING CANNED)
Anchovy
Bass
Bluefish
Catfish
Cod
Flounder
Herring
Monkfish
Red snapper
Salmon
Sardines
Scrod
Sole
Swordfish
Trout
Tuna
Whitefish

SHELLFISH
Clams
Crab
Crawfish
Lobster
Mussels*
Oysters*
Scallops
Shrimp
Squid

EGGS, ANY STYLE

CHEESE†
You may eat 3 to 4 ounces of full-fat firm, soft, and semisoft aged cheeses such as:

Blue
Brie
Camembert
Cream cheese
Cheddar
Feta
Fontina
Goat cheese
Gouda
Gruyère
Havarti
Jarlsburg
Monterey Jack
Mozzarella
Muenster
Parmesan
Provolone
Roman
Sardo
Swiss

†All cheeses have some carbohydrates, and that governs quantities. During Induction, consumption should be limited to 3 to 4 ounces daily. The rule of thumb is to count 1 ounce of cheese as 1 gram of carbohydrate. Fresh cheese, such as cottage cheese and farmer cheese, is too high in carbohydrates for Induction. No diet cheese, cheese spreads, or whey cheeses are allowed in Induction. Those with a known yeast infection, dairy allergy, or cheese intolerance must avoid cheese. Imitation cheese products are not allowed except for soy or rice cheese— but check the carbohydrate content.

*Oysters and mussels are higher in carbs than other shellfish so limit them to 4 ounces a day.

SOY

Soy milk (unsweetened)

Tempeh (fermented soy bean cake)

Tofu (bean curd)

FATS AND OILS*

Butter†

Canola oil

Corn oil

Cream

Flaxseed oil

Grapeseed oil

Half-and-half

Mayonnaise

Olive oil

Safflower oil

Sesame oil

Sour cream

Soybean oil

Sunflower oil

Whipped cream (unsweetened)

*Oils labeled "cold-pressed" or "expeller-pressed" have the most nutrients. Do not cook polyunsaturated oils, such as corn, soybean, and sunflower, at high temperatures or allow them to brown and smoke. Do not heat flaxseed oil.

†Avoid margarine, not because of its carbohydrate content but because it is usually made of trans fats (hydrogenated oils), which pose health risks. (Some nonhydrogenated margarines are available in natural-food stores and selected supermarkets.)

SALAD VEGETABLES

You can have 3 cups (loosely packed) of the following:

Alfalfa sprouts

Arugula

Bean sprouts

Cabbage

Celery

Chicory

Chinese cabbage

Cucumber

Daikon

Endive

Escarole

Fennel

Jicama

Lettuce

Mushrooms

Parsley

Peppers

Radicchio

Radishes

Sorrel

Watercress

For salad dressing, use the desired oil plus vinegar or lemon juice. Commercial brands of salad dressing with fewer than 2 grams of Net Carbs per serving can be used. Small amounts (less than 1 teaspoon per serving) of balsamic vinegar are permissable.

SPICES

Dry granulated spices are allowed as long as they do not contain sugar. If the package refers to unspecified "spices" in addition to the spice you desire, those "spices" may contain sugar, so be careful.

Vegetables in Addition to Salad Vegetables

During the Induction phase, these low carbohydrate vegetables can replace 1 cup of salad.

Artichoke hearts
Asparagus
Bamboo shoots
Beet greens
Bok choy
Broccoli
Broccoli rabe
Brussels sprouts
Cabbage
Cauliflower
Celery root
Collard greens
Dandelion greens
Eggplant
Hearts of Palm
Kale
Kohlrabi
Leeks
Okra
Pumpkin
Rhubarb
Sauerkraut
Scallions
Snow pea pods
Spaghetti squash
Spinach
String beans
Swiss chard
Tomato
Turnips
Water chestnuts
Wax beans
Yellow squash
Zucchini

Herbs and Spices

Basil
Cayenne
Chives
Cilantro
Dill
Garlic
Ginger
Oregano
Pepper
Rosemary
Sage
Tarragon
Thyme

Salad Garnishes

Crumbled crisp bacon
Finely chopped hard-boiled egg yolk
Grated cheese
Onion
Sour cream
Sautéed mushrooms

Beverages

Clear broth/bouillon (not all brands; read the label)
Club soda
Cream, heavy or light (note carbohydrate content)
Decaffeinated coffee or tea*
Essence-flavored seltzer (must say "no calories")
Grain beverages (i.e., imitation coffee substitutes) are not allowed.
Herb tea

*Caffeine should be avoided by those who suspect they are caffeine-dependent and consumed only in limited quantities (perhaps 1 cup a day) by others.

Iced tea sweetened with Splenda®
Mineral water
Spring water
Water

Note: Alcoholic beverages are not part of Induction, but those low in carbohydrates are, in moderation, an option for the later phases of the program.

ARTIFICIAL SWEETENERS

Consumed in moderation, artificial sweeteners make it possible for those trying to lose weight to enjoy the taste of sweets.

Sucralose (marketed as Splenda) is our preferred sweetener; it is the only sweetener made from sugar. It does *not* raise blood sugar, and the Food and Drug Administration approved it in 1998 after reviewing more than one hundred studies. Saccharin (marketed as Sweet'N Low), cyclamate, and acesulfame-K are all acceptable as well.

Remember that each packet of sugar substitute contains about 1 gram of carbohydrate, which must be counted.

Special Category Foods

For variety each day, you can eat 10 to 20 olives, half a small avocado, one ounce of sour cream, or three ounces of unsweetened heavy cream, as well as two to three tablespoons of lemon or lime juice. You may also eat one slice of Atkins Bakery™ Ready-to-Eat Sliced Bread per day, as well as enjoy Atkins Advantage™ Bars and Shakes. A greater variety of Atkins brand and low carb products can be added in later phases. (Be aware that some of these foods occasionally slow down weight loss in some people and may need to be avoided in the first two weeks.) Be sure to count these carbs.

Acceptable Foods for Ongoing Weight Loss

In the second phase of Atkins, *most* people can reintroduce the following foods.

NUTS AND SEEDS*
Almonds
Brazil nuts
Coconut
Hazelnuts (filberts)
Macadamias
Pecans
Pine nuts
Pistachios

Pumpkin seeds
Sesame seeds
Sunflower seeds
Walnuts

*If you stay on Induction more than two weeks, you can add nuts and seeds back into your daily total of 20 grams of Net Carbs.

FRESH CHEESES
Cottage
Farmer
Goat

Mascarpone
Pot cheese
Ricotta

BERRIES
Blackberries
Blueberries

Cranberries
Raspberries
Strawberries

Acceptable Foods for Pre-Maintenance

In this phase, most people can add back the following foods. Add categories in the order listed and introduce only one new food at a time.

DAIRY
Full-fat yogurt, plain*
Whole milk*

NUTS AND SEEDS
Cashews (see Note)
Chestnuts†
Peanuts*

Note: Cashew nuts are technically a fruit and are higher in carbs than other nuts. Peanuts are technically legumes and also higher in carbs than other nuts.

LEGUMES
Black-eyed peas*
Black beans
Chickpeas
Kidney beans
Lentils
Navy beans
Peas, dried/split
Pinto beans*
Soybeans

*Eat in moderation.

†Eat sparingly.

FRUIT OTHER THAN BERRIES
Apple
Apricot*
Banana†
Cherries
Grapefruit
Grapefruit juice
Grapes*
Kiwi*
Mango*
Melon (cantaloupe, crenshaw, honeydew)*
Nectarine*
Orange
Papaya*
Peach
Pear
Pineapple*
Plum
Prunes†
Raisins†
Tangerine
Watermelon*

STARCHY VEGETABLES

- Beets*
- Carrots*
- Corn†
- Peas*
- Pumpkin*
- Sweet potato†
- Potato, white†
- Parsnips†
- Taro*
- Winter squash (acorn, butternut, etc.)
- Yams*
- Yuca*

WHOLE GRAINS

- Amaranth*
- Barley
- Bread, whole wheat/whole-grain*
- Buckwheat*
- Bulgur*
- Cereals, whole-grain†
- Couscous†
- Oatmeal
- Whole wheat pasta

*Eat in moderation.

†Eat sparingly.

ABOUT THE ATKINS
CONTROLLED CARB LIFESTYLE

Want to be up on the latest breakthroughs, news about Atkins, and products that make it easier than ever to eat and cook the controlled carb way?

If you enjoyed *Dr. Atkins' Quick & Easy New Diet Cookbook* (Simon & Schuster) and would like to learn more, you may also want to read:

Dr. Atkins' New Diet Revolution (Avon). The #1 bestselling book that started it all, now revised and updated! Includes new chapters, new recipes, and tips to jump-start weight loss, plus all you need to know to follow this revolutionary weight-loss program.

Atkins for Life (St. Martin's Press). Once you've achieved your goal weight, or have just a few pounds to lose, this Lifetime Maintenance program will allow you to become and remain slim and healthy permanently. Includes 125 recipes and more than six months of meal plans.

Dr. Atkins' New Carbohydrate Gram Counter (M. Evans). This completely updated and expanded edition introduces the concept of Net Carbs, the only carbs you need to count when you do Atkins, a fast-food section, and many other features.

The Atkins Journal (M. Evans). This 120-day journal helps you record your meals and snacks, track your weight loss, and deal with issues you may confront on the journey to a new you. Includes weekly pages for weighing in, rating your progress, and recording your feelings.

Dr. Atkins' Age-Defying Diet Revolution (St. Martin's Press). Eat well and stay young! Thirty years of Dr. Atkins' experience with nutrition and the latest scientific breakthroughs lead to his new, stay-younger-longer regimen. Using this simple program you can defy your age and extend your life!

Dr. Atkins' Vita-Nutrient Solution (Simon & Schuster). A comprehensive guide to more than 120 supplements, including vitamins, minerals, antioxidants, amino acids, and herbs. An indispensable resource for anyone who wants a natural approach to health and well-being.

Atkins Nutritionals, Inc., makes a full line of low carbohydrate alternative foods and ingredients. Many of them are listed below.

Atkins Advantage™ Shake Mix in Strawberry,* Chocolate, Vanilla, and Cappuccino

Atkins Quick Quisine™ Bake Mix*

Atkins Quick Quisine™ Pancake & Waffle Mix*

Atkins Quick Quisine™ Lemon Poppy Bake Mix*

Atkins Quick Quisine™ Orange Cranberry Bake Mix

Atkins Quick Quisine™ Banana Nut Bake Mix

Atkins Quick Quisine™ Chocolate Chocolate Chip Bake Mix

Atkins Kitchen™ Quick & Easy Bread Mix in Country White,* Sourdough, and Caraway Rye

Atkins Bakery™ Ready-to-Eat Sliced Bread in White,* Rye, and Multigrain

Atkins Bakery™ Freeze N' Thaw Bread

Atkins Quick Quisine™ Sugar Free Pancake Syrup*

Atkins™ Sugar Free Syrup in Caramel, Raspberry, Chocolate, and Strawberry

Atkins Quick Quisine™ Ketch-A-Tomato*

Atkins Quick Quisine™ Barbeque Sauce*

Atkins Quick Quisine™ Steak Sauce

Atkins Quick Quisine™ Teriyaki Sauce

Atkins Quick Quisine™ Pasta Cuts in Penne,* Orzo, Spaghetti, Cut Fettuccine, and Fusilli

Atkins Quick Quisine™ Pasta Sides

Atkins Endulge™ Chocolate Candy Bars

Atkins Endulge™ Ice Cream*

Atkins Morning Start™ Bars

Atkins Morning Start™ Ready-to-Eat Cereals

Atkins Bakery™ Bagels

All these and other Atkins products can be ordered from www.atkins.com. For a local retailer, go to the Retail Locator on the Web site or call 1-800-2-ATKINS.

*Used in recipes in this book

ABOUT THE AUTHORS

ROBERT C. ATKINS, M.D., was the founder and medical director of the Atkins Center for Complementary Medicine and the founder of the Dr. Robert C. Atkins Foundation. A 1951 graduate of the University of Michigan, he received his medical degree from Cornell University Medical School in 1955 and went on to specialize in cardiology. He was a practicing physician for more than forty years and is the author of more than a dozen books. As a leader in the areas of natural medicine and nutritional pharmacology, he built an international reputation. He was the recipient of the World Organization of Alternative Medicine's Recognition of Achievement Award and the National Health Federation's Man of the Year. His many media appearances, where he discussed diet and health, included *Larry King Live, Oprah, CBS This Morning,* and *CNBC,* among others. Many magazine and newspaper articles have featured his work, and he also had a nationally syndicated radio show. For many years Dr. Atkins was the editor of his own national monthly newsletter, "Dr. Atkins' Health Revelations," which was followed by a similar electronic newsletter. He died after sustaining injuries in a fall in April 2003.

VERONICA ATKINS was born in Russia and narrowly escaped the Nazi onslaught during World War II by fleeing to Vienna, where she lived with her great aunt. In the years since, she has lived in seven countries and become fluent in as many languages. Her far-flung travels have given her an extensive knowledge of international cuisine. Music has also played an important role in her life. She began singing in Europe at a young age and performed professionally as an opera singer from 1963 to 1976. Today she is actively involved in extending Dr. Atkins' legacy through the Dr. Robert C. Atkins Foundation. She also serves on the board of directors of the Foundation for the Advancement of Innovative Medicine Education Group. Her current stage is the kitchen, where she actively creates and develops delicious controlled carbohydrate recipes.